God says Yes, We say Amen

HE HEALS TODAY!

HEALING FOR YOUR BODY, SOUL, AND SPIRIT
- A BIBLE STUDY -

BY CINDY COX

Unless otherwise indicated, all Scripture quotations are taken from the *New King James Version* of the Bible. Copyright © 1982 by Thomas Nelson, Inc. Used by permission. All rights reserved.

Scripture quotations marked AMP are taken from the *Amplified Bible* copyright © 1954, 1958, 1962, 1964, 1965, 1987 by the Lockman Foundation. All rights reserved. Used by permission.

Scripture quotations marked NIV are taken from *The Holy Bible: New International Version*. Copyright © 1973, 1978, 1984 by the International Bible Society. Used by permission of Zondervan Bible Publishers. All rights reserved.

Scripture quotations marked The Message are taken from THE MESSAGE, copyright © 1993, 1994, 1995, 1996, 2000, 2001, 2002. Used by permission of NavPress Publishing Group.

Scripture quotations marked NLT are taken from *The Holy Bible, New Living Translation*, copyright © 1996, 2004. Use by permission of Tyndale House Publishers, Inc., Wheaton, Illinois 60189. All rights reserved.

All direct Scripture quotations are noted in italic print. Any bold highlights or underlines were added by the author for emphasis.

God Says Yes, We Say Amen
ISBN 978-0-9906802-0-8
Copyright © 2015 by
Cindy Cox

Published by
Christian Illness Support, LLC
14418 Knightsbridge Dr.
Shelby Twp., MI 48315
www.JesusChristHealsToday.com
Email: info@JesusChristHealsToday.com

Graphic Layout & Cover Design: Keigh Cox

Printed in the United States of America. All rights reserved under International Copyright Law. Contents and/or cover may not be reproduced in whole or in part in any form without the express written consent of the publisher.

DISCLAIMER - As ambassadors of Christ and ministers of healing, we are not responsible for a person's disease, nor are we responsible for their healing. We simply share God's Word and what He says about this subject. There is no guarantee that any person will be healed or any disease be prevented. The fruits of this ministry will come forth out of the relationship between the person and God based on their knowledge, belief, and application of revelation of His perfect will.

DEDICATION

To Kent, my husband, my best friend, my strength.
Your love for me, your affirmation, and your support are the wind beneath my wings.
Without you, I wouldn't be me!
Your amazing gifts are a treasure in the Kingdom of God, rich beyond compare.
Others may not see.
Others may not notice.
But God sees, and He is well pleased!

To Pastor Tim McCarthy, my mentor, my spiritual father.
I was hungry, and you fed me. I was thirsty and you gave me something to drink.
You have taught me, encouraged me, and sent me out with your blessing and His
to bring heaven to earth!
I deeply love and appreciate you and your beautiful wife, Fran!

And to Jesus, my Healer, my Redeemer, the Love of my life!
I live in awe of You.
I believe, therefore I receive --
All of You
All that you lived and died to freely give.

And I freely give You all of me!
With joy!!!

ACKNOWLEDGEMENTS

Thank you to Kent, my amazing husband. You help me more than I can begin to acknowledge here! I stand in awe of how God paired us up so perfectly. You fill in my "blanks" and I fill in yours! Together, we're a whole. Thank you for taking care of every detail of the technology and administrative needs of this God idea! Thank you for listening to me and talking with me, supporting me 100%, and loving me always and forever! I truly am the most blessed woman in the world to have you for my husband!

Thank you to Keigh, our amazing daughter-in-law, and my spiritual daughter. Your gifts continue to bless us, and to bless the Kingdom of God. Your artwork and graphic layout of *God Says Yes, We Say Amen* are truly Holy Spirit inspired! Thank you for offering your precious time and talent to the Lord and to His people! I love you, sweet daughter!

Thank you to Denise Baum, my friend and sister in Christ. We share one mind, one heart, one passion … Jesus! Thank you for reading this Bible study and providing invaluable feedback and affirmation of the Holy Spirit's mighty move upon and through it. You are a treasure. God even says so in His Word! In 2 Corinthians 4:7, He says, *But we have this treasure in earthen vessels, that the excellence of the power may be of God and not of us.* He works through you, girlfriend! You are His treasure and mine!!!

Most of all, thank you Father God. Thank you for calling me and anointing me to carry forth Your message of truth to the nations. May You be blessed, Lord, as Your kids receive Your indescribable, inexpressible, free Gift!

CONTENTS

INTRODUCTION:

   Introduction   9

   Notes to the Participant   10

   Notes to the Leader   11

BIBLE STUDY SESSIONS:

   Session 1: Yes, It IS God's Will to Heal!   15

   Session 2: God's Perfect Will for You!   27

   Session 3: Faith … Simply Believe   43

   Session 4: Great Faith   55

   Session 5: Positioned to Receive   67

   Session 6: Seek the Healer   79

   Session 7: Godly Living   93

   Session 8: Forgive, As You Have Been Forgiven   107

   Session 9: Jesus, Healer of the Wounded Soul   121

   Session 10: Fear Not, Only Believe   139

EXTRAS:

   Questions and Answers   155

   Index   177

   Receiving Salvation   179

   Receiving Baptism of the Holy Spirit   180

   God's Medicine: Declarations for Healing and Divine Health   181

   Also by Cindy Cox   185

   Contact and Ordering Information   188

INTRODUCTION

For all of God's promises have been fulfilled in Christ with a resounding "Yes!" And through Christ, our "Amen" (which means "Yes") ascends to God for his glory.

2 Corinthians 1:20 NLT

I was diagnosed with Stage 4 melanoma in February of 2002. The cancer had metastasized throughout my lymphatic system. It was considered incurable, and my life expectancy without medical intervention was 6 to 9 months.

At the time of my diagnosis, I didn't have any knowledge of Jesus the Healer. In fact, I didn't even know Jesus as my Lord and my Savior. But I was introduced to God's promises through Jenn, a precious friend and woman of God, and began my journey of healing. Six months after receiving Jesus into my life as my Lord, my Savior, and my Healer, I was declared free from cancer … without ANY MEDICAL INTERVENTION!

So many people have asked me, "What did you do to receive your healing?" The answer is really quite simple. I learned what God's promises of healing are, according to His Word. I received His truth into my heart. I believed. He said "Yes"! I said "Amen"!

In the years since my healing, my husband Kent and I have shared these same amazing promises with countless people across the world, through face to face teaching and prayer, through our books, our website, and our video and audio podcasts. And we have seen countless people receive healing and so very much more from Abba Father. My burning passion is to take God's message of healing to the world. This Bible study was consummated through intimate relationship with my Father, conceived in my heart, and birthed in this very study that is in your hands.

With all my heart, I believe that as God's promises are revealed to you, the seed of His Word will take root in your heart, and produce the precious fruit of healing! And our God will be glorified!!!

In His Love and Abundant Blessings,

Cindy Cox
Author and Teacher

God Says Yes, We Say Amen
He Heals Today!
Healing for Your Body, Soul, and Spirit – A Bible Study

NOTES TO THE PARTICIPANT
How to get the most out of this Bible Study.

God Says Yes, We Say Amen was designed to be used within a 10-week small group or healing school setting. Each participant should have his/her own Bible study guide in order to benefit richly from the in-depth study session and follow up reading.

Each session begins with a Session Purpose; an overview of the teaching.
- Sessions 1 and 2 lay the biblical groundwork of God's perfect will to heal, always! God says, "Yes"!
- Sessions 3, 4, and 5 reveal our only requirement in receiving … to believe! We say, "Amen"!
- Session 6 is a pivotal lesson that teaches how to develop a true relationship with God. How can we possibly believe God's will to heal if we don't know Him and trust Him?
- In Sessions 7 through 10, deceptive tactics of the enemy are exposed that may hinder our believing and receiving. You will learn to overcome those deceptions using your authority and power as a believer!

Each Session is broken into Foundations, or "big ideas". You'll notice lots of Scripture references and open-ended questions and statements within each Foundation. This is an inductive Bible study, supplying biblical evidence regarding God's grace and His will to heal. As you feed your heart with His promises, He will reveal His will to you through His Word!

There is a Question and Answer section in the back of this workbook to guide your study if needed.

Following each study session, there is an application opportunity titled, Keeping God's Word … Receiving It, Loving It, Living It. It is critically important that we do not merely listen to the Word, and so deceive ourselves. We are instructed to do what it says. (James 1:22) As you hear the Word, receive it openly, treasure it in within your heart, and then live it … the seed sown will produce a great harvest! (Matthew 13:23)

The third segment of each week's session is titled, In Pursuit of More. This is more than a "bonus" or "extra credit". DO NOT SKIP OVER THIS SECTION!!! It is pure manna from God's Word … deep and powerful truth that has the potential to set you free! Take the time during the week to read and reread this section. Take time to talk to God about your thinking, your questions, your new understandings. Let Him speak to you through His Word as you review scriptures from the session. Let Him stir up your hunger for Him and His truth.

NOTES TO THE LEADER

Preparation
Thank you for your commitment to lead this study group! As the leader of this small group healing ministry, you are an ambassador for Christ, sharing the Good News of healing as you lead others through *God Says Yes, We Say Amen*. Please take ample time before each session to watch the teaching DVD, and to read each session in full, taking time to meditate on the scriptures referenced. Complete your own workbook before each lesson to help guide discussion and answer questions. There is a <u>Question and Answer</u> section in the back of this workbook for your support.

My prayer is that the God of our Lord Jesus Christ, the glorious Father, may give you the Spirit of wisdom and revelation as you prepare for and lead this Bible study. (Ephesians 1:17)

Scheduling and Needs
Schedule a two-hour block of time for each session in order to give adequate time to the people to take in and process the teaching presented. I suggest opening each session with prayer and an opportunity to share testimonies (about 15 minutes). Watch the teaching DVD together, completing the open-ended questions and statements in the workbook in the process (about 60 minutes). After viewing the DVD together, allow time for questions and discussion (about 30 minutes). Close with corporate healing prayer, and/or individual prayer and guidance (about 15 minutes).

It is important that each person has his/her own copy of the *God Says Yes, We Say Amen* Bible study guide. They will use it during the small-group session, and throughout the week as they meditate on God's truth presented during that week's meeting. The follow-up section, <u>Keeping God's Word ... Receiving It, Loving It, Living It</u> leads the people to apply God's Word into their life. And as they read the section, <u>In Pursuit of More</u>, the completeness of God's perfect will to heal will become even more firmly established in their heart!

Session DVDs
A set of teaching DVDs is included in your Leader's Kit of *God says Yes, We Say Amen*. Each teaching is about 1 hour in length, and delves deep into that session's topic, unveiling the overwhelming richness of God's truth. Be prepared with the technical equipment and support needed in order to view the session DVD.

Prayer Support
Allow the Holy Spirit to lead you as you lead this study. Pray corporately. Pray individually. Pray fervently. Pray with the authority you have as a believing believer! More people are healed when we pray for more people! *Heal the sick, cleanse the lepers, raise the dead! Freely you have received, freely give!* (Matthew 10:8)

Consider supplying those in your small group with your personal contact information, in order that they can call you with questions or for prayer needs during the week. Discipleship requires investment. Investment results in a great harvest!

Questions/Celebrations
Please contact me by email with questions that come up that may be difficult to address, and with the outpouring of healing testimonies that will surely result from this study!

info@cindycoxministries.com

May you be abundantly blessed through your giving!

In His love,
Cindy

YES, IT IS GOD'S WILL TO HEAL!

...and by His stripes you are healed.
Isaiah 53:5

SESSION 1

16 GOD SAYS YES, WE SAY AMEN

> ## SESSION PURPOSE
>
> How often have we heard the phrase, "If it be God's will" in conjunction with healing? The purpose of this study session is to settle once and for all, that there is no IF in God's will to heal. Eternal salvation and healing of the physical body go hand in hand and should never be separated. Let's look to the Word of God to explain …

Foundation One

In this section, you will study 3 foundational pieces of scriptural evidence that **it is God's will to heal!**

Scriptural Evidence #1: Isaiah 53:4-5
Isaiah prophesied the coming of our Redeemer 700 years before His birth!

> *Surely He has borne our <u>griefs</u>*
> *And carried our <u>sorrows</u>;*
> *Yet we esteemed Him stricken,*
> *Smitten by God, and afflicted.*
> *But He was wounded for our <u>transgressions</u>,*
> *He was bruised for our <u>iniquities</u>;*
> *The <u>chastisement</u> for our <u>peace</u> was upon Him,*
> *And by His stripes we are <u>healed</u>.*

Word study: The Old Testament was written in the Hebrew language. The words that are underlined in the Isaiah scripture above have very rich, deep meaning, that isn't adequately translated into English. If you look these words up in a <u>Strong's Concordance</u> (Hebrew numbers and words are included below), you'll uncover layers of meaning that reveal God's will to heal! You may want to do this word study on your own! You can access an easy-to-use concordance at http://www.eliyah.com/lexicon.html.

Write the meanings of the following words:

1. Griefs (H2483 – *choliy*) [handwritten: Total 24x — sickness (12x), disease (7x), grief (4x), sick (1x). from H2470: malady, anxiety, calamity; -disease, grief, is sick(ness)]

2. Sorrows (H4341 – *mak'ob*) [handwritten: 1. pain sorrow a. pain (physical) b. pain (mental)]

YES, IT IS GOD'S WILL TO HEAL! 17

3. Transgressions (H6588 – *pesha/pasha*), trespass (5x), sin (3x), rebellion (1x) a revolt (national, moral or religious) - rebellion, sin, transgression, trespass

4. Iniquities (H5771 – *'avon*) perversity, ie. (moral) evil: -fault, iniquity, mischief, punishment (of iniquity), sin.

5. Chastisement (H4148 – *muwcar*) figuratively, reproof, warning or instruction; also restraint: -bond, chastening (eth), check, correction, discipline, doctrine, instruction, rebuke.

6. Peace (H7965 – *shalowm*) well, peaceably, welfare, salute, prosperity, did, safe, health, peaceable. Completeness (in number), safety, soundness (in body) tranquility, contentment, peace, friendship; w/ God, covenant, w/ human, peace from war, peace as adjective.

7. Healed (H7495 – *rapha*) KJV: heal, physician, cure, repaired [(seizing & plucking (chaldee Lexicon)] Premative root; properly, to mend (by stitching), ie. (figuratively) to cure, heal, thoroughly, make whole.

The Hebrew word *rapha* is actually one of the names of God – Jehovah Rapha – God Who Heals! Often times this word is misinterpreted to mean spiritual healing only. But that is simply not the full meaning of the Hebrew word. *Rapha* is used 67 times in the Old Testament, and it is translated "heal" 57 times! Here are a few examples of Scriptures using the Hebrew word *rapha*:

2 Kings 20:5-6
"Return and tell Hezekiah the leader of My people, 'Thus says the Lord, the God of David your father: "I have heard your prayer, I have seen your tears; surely I will **heal** you. On the third day you shall go up to the house of the Lord. And I will add to your days fifteen years. I will deliver you and this city from the hand of the king of Assyria; and I will defend this city for My own sake, and for the sake of My servant David."'

heal - for Gods purpose

Psalm 103:1-5
Bless the Lord, O my soul;
And all that is within me, bless His holy name!
Bless the Lord, O my soul,
And forget not all His benefits:
Who forgives all your iniquities,
Who **heals** all your diseases,
Who redeems your life from destruction,
Who crowns you with lovingkindness and tender mercies,
Who satisfies your mouth with good things,
So that your youth is renewed like the eagle's.

Psalm 147:3
He **heals** the brokenhearted and binds up all their wounds.

Now, read and soak in the following paraphrase of Isaiah 53:4-5 that unveils God's great promise for His children!

> *Surely He has borne our sickness and disease, and carried our mental and physical pain; yet we esteemed Him stricken, smitten by God, and afflicted. But He was wounded for our unknown sins. He was bruised for our willful disobedience. The penalty, the cost, for our complete wholeness was upon Him; and by His stripes we are healed – spirit, soul, and body!*

***

Scriptural Evidence #2: Matthew 8:16-17
Isaiah's prophetic word was fulfilled by Jesus, through His ministry on this earth. A fulfilled prophecy means that the prophecy was verified, that the prediction was completed!

> *When evening had come, they brought to Him many who were demon-possessed. And he cast out the spirits with His words, and healed all who were sick, that it might be fulfilled which was spoken by Isaiah the prophet saying: "He Himself took our infirmities and bore our sicknesses."*

8. How many were brought to Jesus?
   Many

9. How many did He heal?
   All who where sick

10. What was the ultimate purpose for His healing? *It might be fulfilled which was spoken by Isaiah the prophet* — prophecy

Write the meanings of the following words:

11. Took (G2983 – *lambanō*)
    receive, take, have, catch,

12. Infirmities (G769 – *astheneia*)
    feebleness (of mind or body); by implication, malady; morally, frailty – disease, infirmity, sickness, weakness

13. Bore (G941 – *bastazō*)
    (through the idea of removal); to lift, literally or figuratively (endure, declare, sustain, receive, etc.) bear, carry, take up

Jesus took our weaknesses of body and soul in order to carry them away! He bore our sicknesses upon Himself, in order to bear our burdens for us! Therefore we do NOT need to carry them ourselves! He paid the price in full for our complete wholeness!

***

Scriptural Evidence #3: 1 Peter 2:24
After Jesus had died as our Sacrificial Lamb, and had been raised as our Great Redeemer, the apostles went on to preach this amazing news about Jesus, our Healer!

> *who Himself bore our sins in His own body on the tree, that we, having died to sins, might live for righteousness – by whose stripes you were <u>healed</u>.*

Forgiveness of sin and healing of the <u>soul</u> and <u>body</u> are directly connected, just as they are in this God-breathed scripture! Jesus bore our sins in His own body when He was crucified. Our debt was canceled out when He paid the penalty for us. But here's an amazing thought … Jesus took the stripes on His holy back <u>before</u> He carried our sin to the cross. He paid for our healing <u>before</u> He paid for our sin!

14. When did we die to sin and gain access to a life of righteousness?

When Jesus healed us then came freedom of sin.

15. What is the meaning of the word "healed" (G2390 – *iaomai*)? *Make whole, heal, make whole.*

The Greek word <u>*iaomai*</u> clearly refers to <u>physical healing</u>. It is used 28 times in the New Testament. Here are 3 examples!

Matthew 8:8, 13
> *The centurion answered and said, "Lord, I am not worthy that You should come under my roof. But only speak a word, and my servant will be <u>healed</u>. Then Jesus said to the centurion, "Go your way; and as you have believed, so let it be done for you." And his servant was <u>healed</u> that same hour.*

= selfless

Mark 5:29
> *Immediately the fountain of her blood was dried up, and <u>she felt</u> in her body that she was <u>healed</u> of the affliction.*

Luke 22:50-51
> *And one of them struck the servant of the high priest and cut off his right ear. But Jesus answered and said, "Permit even this." And He touched his ear and <u>healed</u> him.*

Righting peters wrong.

[Handwritten margin note: Healed — Hebrew: rapha, Greek: iaomaia]

Foundation Two

[Healing is part of salvation!]

There is an amazing Greek word used 110 times in the New Testament – *sozo*. The depth of this word is vast, encompassing all that salvation brings to an individual. *Sozo* refers to the entire provision of God for the whole man – his spirit, his soul, and his body.

Read the following scriptures, highlighting the words save, saved, healed, made well, or made whole in each scripture. Know that each of these words is the very same original Greek word – *sozo* – the entire provision of God for the whole man – spirit, soul and body!

Sozo includes salvation for man's spirit, including forgiveness and eternal life!

    Matthew 1:21 *[handwritten: his people from their sins]*

    Luke 19:9-10

    John 3:16-17

    Acts 16:30-31

    Romans 10:9

    1 Timothy 2:3-4

Sozo includes healing for man's body!

    Mark 5:22-23 *[handwritten: come & lay your hands]*

    Luke 18:41-42

    Acts 14:8-10

Sozo includes healing for man's soul (deliverance)!

    Luke 8:33-36

Sozo includes being made whole!

    Matthew 9:21-22

    Luke 17:12-19

    Acts 4:9-12

༄༅ ༄༅

Final thought …

Ephesians 2:8 says, *For by grace you have been saved through faith, and that not of yourselves; it is the gift of God.*

The word "saved" in this scripture, once again, is *sozo*. *Sozo*, according to God's Word, includes salvation, healing, deliverance, and being made whole. Therefore …

> *… by grace you have been saved, healed, delivered, and made whole through faith, and that not of yourselves; it is the gift of God!*

KEEPING GOD'S WORD
Receiving It, Loving It, Living It

1. Meditate on this scriptural truth daily!

   Surely, Jesus has borne my sickness and carried my pain.
   Therefore I don't need to carry it! By His stripes I have been healed!

2. Envision yourself totally healed, head to toe.

3. Write a journal entry about something you envision yourself doing in your healthy body, mind, or relationship!

IN PURSUIT OF MORE

I Received Salvation … I Received Healing

February 19, 2002 was the day that I received my salvation. I had been diagnosed with stage-four melanoma 6 days earlier. The cancer was considered incurable according to medical expertise. My life prognosis was 6 to 9 months. I was consumed with indescribable fear and dread of what was to come as the disease progressed. Symptoms – pain and abdominal masses – appeared within days of the diagnosis.

A young teacher in the school in which I taught offered me a glimmer of light during this dark time in my life. She shared with me the truth that Jesus paid the price for my healing at the same time that He paid the price for my forgiveness and salvation. This was new news to me, something I had never heard before.

Then she led me in a prayer of salvation. A prayer of surrender to my Savior. A prayer that opened heaven's gates wide to God's grace for me! A prayer that signed and sealed my adoption as Abba Father's child! A prayer that gave me the right to my inheritance of the Kingdom of God!

Six months later, I was completely healed of the melanoma. I had no chemotherapy. I had no radiation. I received the healing Jesus provided for me when He took the stripes on His holy back. I received salvation!

Forgiveness AND Healing are Part of Salvation

Let's take a close look at scriptural evidence that healing of your body is directly related to forgiveness of your sins through salvation!

1 Peter 2:24
> *who Himself bore our sins in His own body on the tree, that we, having died to sins, might live for righteousness—by whose stripes you were healed.*

In this scripture, there are 2 distinct sentence clauses. The first clause illuminates the truth that Jesus, our Savior, took our sins upon His own body for the purpose of purchasing our righteousness. When we receive salvation through faith in Jesus, it is as if we were crucified with Jesus, and resurrected to new life. The old is gone, and we become brand new! Cleansed from sin through the shed blood of Jesus!

But that's not all! Notice the second clause in this scripture, separated from the first clause by a dash. (In the Old King James translation, a colon is used here.) The correct grammatical use of a colon or a dash is to connect two clauses when the second clause strongly relates back to the first clause. Before Jesus was crucified, He was whipped. That whip tore stripes into His holy flesh in order to provide for your healing! His body was broken and bruised so yours could be whole and healed! His passion, crucifixion and resurrection made the way for your healing, your forgiveness, your salvation! Selah! Stop and think about that! May Jesus be exalted and lifted high!

James 5:14-15
> *Is anyone among you sick? Let him call for the elders of the church, and let them pray over him, anointing him with <u>oil</u> in the <u>name of the Lord</u>. And the <u>prayer of faith will save</u> the sick, and the Lord will raise him up. And if he has committed sins, he will be forgiven.*

The word <u>save</u> in this scripture is once again the Greek word *sozo*. God tells us in His Word that the prayer of faith will *sozo* the sick. Remember that the word *sozo* means to save, to heal, to deliver, to make whole. While the NKJV translation of James 5:15 says: *the prayer of faith will <u>save the sick</u>*, the NIV translation of James 5:15 says: *the prayer offered in faith <u>will make the sick person well</u>*.

Take another look at this scripture:
> *Is anyone among you sick? Let him call for the elders of the church, <u>and</u> let them pray over him, anointing him with oil in the name of the Lord. <u>And</u> the prayer of faith will save the sick, <u>and</u> the Lord will raise him up. <u>And</u> if he has committed sins, he will be forgiven.*

The conjunction "and" is used <u>4 times in</u> <u>these 2 verses</u>! As a writer, I would try to avoid using that word so frequently. But the conjunction "and" serves a purpose. It joins together related ideas. All of the following streams of grace are connected – perhaps that's why the conjunction "and" was used 4 times in this scripture!

Call the elders (believing believers) to pray for you with fervency, anointing you with oil…
- And the prayer of faith will <u>save the sick</u>, (save, heal, deliver, make whole)
- And the Lord will <u>raise him up</u>. (to arouse from the sleep of death, to recall the dead to life)
- And if he has committed sins, <u>he will be forgiven</u>. (remission of sin)

Luke 5:18-26

Then behold, men brought on a bed a man who was paralyzed, whom they sought to bring in and lay before Him. And when they could not find how they might bring him in, because of the crowd, they went up on the housetop and let him down with his bed through the tiling into the midst before Jesus.

When He saw their faith, He said to him, "Man, your sins are forgiven you."

And the scribes and the Pharisees began to reason, saying, "Who is this who speaks blasphemies? Who can forgive sins but God alone?"

But when Jesus perceived their thoughts, He answered and said to them, "Why are you reasoning in your hearts? Which is easier, to say, 'Your sins are forgiven you,' or to say, 'Rise up and walk'? But that you may know that the Son of Man has power on earth to forgive sins"—He said to the man who was paralyzed, "I say to you, arise, take up your bed, and go to your house."

Immediately he rose up before them, took up what he had been lying on, and departed to his own house, glorifying God. And they were all amazed, and they glorified God and were filled with fear, saying, "We have seen strange things today!"

In this biblical account, when Jesus saw the paralyzed man, He recognized the man's faith and the faith of his friends. Jesus' response was a declaration of forgiveness for the paralyzed man's sin. This caused an uprising among the scribes and Pharisees who began to reason. They began to think about Jesus' statement and then form conclusions and make judgments about Him. *"Who is this who speaks blasphemies? Who can forgive sins but God alone?"*

Look closely at how Jesus responded. He said, *"Which is easier, to say 'Your sins are forgiven you,' or to say, 'Rise up and walk'?"* Then Jesus explained the reason for the choice of his declaration. He said, "Your sins are forgiven you" <u>so that we may know that the Son of Man has power on earth to forgive sins.</u>

Healing of paralysis is clearly visible, isn't it? But forgiveness of sins is not. Jesus brought the invisible into visibility through the physical healing of the man. With the healing that manifested, and with the words Jesus spoke, He showed the heart and the will of God … forgiveness of sins AND healing of the body. Once again, there is a direct connection … because both healing and forgiveness flow in the streams of God's grace!

Psalm 103:1-5

Bless the Lord, O my soul;
And all that is within me, bless His holy name!
Bless the Lord, O my soul,
And forget not all His benefits:
Who forgives all your iniquities,
Who heals all your diseases,
Who redeems your life from destruction,
Who crowns you with lovingkindness and tender mercies,
Who satisfies your mouth with good things,
So that your youth is renewed like the eagle's.

I love this Psalm. I meditate on it frequently to recount the amazing benefits God has provided for me. Once again, forgiveness of sin, physical healing, and salvation are all included and connected in this scripture. I choose to bless the Lord with all my heart, with all that is deep within me, and praise Him for His ultimate, perfect Gift!

※

February 19, 2002 was the day that I received my salvation into the newness of life, the abundance of life that Jesus came to provide. On that day my story changed from death to life! I am saved. I am forgiven. I am healed. I am well … very well!!!

Have you surrendered all to the Lord Jesus? Have you received Him as your Savior? Have you given Him Lordship over all facets of your life? Please pray this prayer with me:

Jesus, I believe in you. I believe that you lived for me, you died for me, and you were resurrected from the dead to provide "sozo" for me! Come into my life, make all the old things new, all the dead things alive. I want your complete wholeness in my life: body, mind and spirit!

GOD'S PERFECT WILL FOR YOU

Jesus Christ is the same yesterday, today, and forever.

Hebrews 13:8

SESSION 2

SESSION PURPOSE

In Session 1, we established the biblical foundation that it truly IS God's will that you are healed. Today we will look at the life of Jesus, and numerous gospel accounts of healing that reveal the heart of the Father and confirm His will to heal.

Herein lies a problem. The sickness and pain that we see in this world contradicts the heart of God. In this lesson, we will explore the difficult question -- Why? We will look at the difference between God's perfect will and His permissive will. We will explore and expose several causes of sickness and disease in this world.

Foundation One

God's perfect will to heal is evidenced through Jesus. We look into the ministry of Jesus to see God's perfect will working through His Son!

In the gospels, there are 23 accounts of Jesus healing specific individuals. Note that these biblical accounts included physical, emotional, and spiritual healings … another piece of evidence that God wants us whole! Take time during the coming weeks to feed on these testimonies of Jesus. As you do, you will come to know His compassion, His love, His desire to take care of you. Your faith will be stirred to rise up and personally encounter the Healer!

1. Royal official's son: John 4:46-54
2. Demon-possessed man in Capernaum: Mark 1:21-28; Luke 4:33-37
3. Peter's mother-in-law: Matthew 8:14-15; Mark 1:29-31; Luke 4:38-39
4. Man with leprosy: Matthew 8:1-3; Mark 1:40-42
5. Centurion's servant: Matthew 8:5-13; Luke 7:1-10
6. Paralyzed man: Matthew 9:1-8; Mark 2:1-12; Luke 5:18-26
7. Man with withered hand: Matthew 12:9-14; Mark 3:1-6; Luke 6:6-10
8. Gerasene demon-possessed man: Matthew 8:28-32; Mark 5:1-13; Luke 8:26-33
9. Woman with issue of blood: Matthew 9:20-22; Mark 5:25-34; Luke 8:43-48
10. Two blind men: Matthew 9:27-31
11. Mute, demon-possessed man: Matthew 9:32-33
12. Man crippled 38 years: John 5:1-15
13. Demon-possessed girl: Matthew 15:21-28; Mark 7:24-30
14. Deaf man: Mark 7:31-37
15. Blind man from Bethsaida: Mark 8:22-26
16. Man born blind: John 9:1-41
17. Demon-possessed boy: Matthew 17:14-20; Mark 9:17-29; Luke 9:37-42
18. Blind and mute demon-possessed man: Matthew 12:22-23; Luke 11:14

19. Woman with 18 year infirmity: Luke 13:10-13
20. Man with dropsy: Luke 14:1-6
21. Ten lepers: Luke 17:11-19
22. Blind Bartimaeus: Matthew 20:29-34; Mark 10:46-52; Luke 18:35-43
23. Restoring the servant of the high priest's severed ear: Luke 22:47-51

In addition to the accounts of Jesus healing specific people with specific needs, there are 17 biblical accounts of Jesus healing <u>all who were in need</u> within a mass of people. Read the following 17 scriptures, and underline the words "all", "every", "many" and "multitude" as you read. Be prepared for God to open your eyes anew and settle His perfect will to heal firmly in your heart!

1. **Matthew 4:23** *And Jesus went about all Galilee, teaching in their synagogues, preaching the gospel of the kingdom, and healing all kinds of sickness and all kinds of disease among the people.*

2. **Matthew 4:24** *Then His fame went throughout all Syria; and they brought to Him all sick people who were afflicted with various diseases and torments, and those who were demon-possessed, epileptics, and paralytics; and He healed them.*

3. **Matthew 8:16** *When evening had come, they brought to Him many who were demon-possessed. And He cast out the spirits with a word, and healed all who were sick,*

4. **Matthew 9:35** *Then Jesus went about all the cities and villages, teaching in their synagogues, preaching the gospel of the kingdom, and healing every sickness and every disease among the people.*

5. **Matthew 12:15** *But when Jesus knew it, He withdrew from there. And great multitudes followed Him, and He healed them all.*

6. **Matthew 14:14** *And when Jesus went out He saw a great multitude; and He was moved with compassion for them, and healed their sick.*

7. **Matthew 14:34-36** *When they had crossed over, they came to the land of Gennesaret. And when the men of that place recognized Him, they sent out into all that surrounding region, brought to Him all who were sick, and begged Him that they might only touch the hem of His garment. And as many as touched it were made perfectly well.*

8. **Matthew 15:30-31** *Then great multitudes came to Him, having with them the lame, blind, mute, maimed, and many others; and they laid them down at Jesus' feet, and He healed them. So the multitude marveled when they saw the mute speaking, the maimed made whole, the lame walking, and the blind seeing; and they glorified the God of Israel.*

9. **Matthew 19:2** *And great multitudes followed Him, and He healed them there.*

10. **Matthew 21:14** *Then the blind and the lame came to Him in the temple, and He healed them.*

11. **Mark 1:32-34** *At evening, when the sun had set, they brought to Him all who were sick and those who were demon-possessed. And the whole city was gathered together at the door. Then He healed many who were sick with various diseases, and cast out many demons; and He did not allow the demons to speak, because they knew Him.*

12. **Mark 3:9-10** *So He told His disciples that a small boat should be kept ready for Him because of the multitude, lest they should crush Him. For He healed many, so that as many as had afflictions pressed about Him to touch Him.*

13. **Mark 6:56** *Wherever He entered, into villages, cities, or the country, they laid the sick in the marketplaces, and begged Him that they might just touch the hem of His garment. And as many as touched Him were made well.*

14. **Luke 4:40** *When the sun was setting, all those who had any that were sick with various diseases brought them to Him; and He laid His hands on every one of them and healed them.*

15. **Luke 6:17-19** *And He came down with them and stood on a level place with a crowd of His disciples and a great multitude of people from all Judea and Jerusalem, and from the seacoast of Tyre and Sidon, who came to hear Him and be healed of their diseases, as well as those who were tormented with unclean spirits. And they were healed. And the whole multitude sought to touch Him, for power went out from Him and healed them all.*

16. **Luke 7:21** *And that very hour He cured many of infirmities, afflictions, and evil spirits; and to many blind He gave sight.*

17. **Luke 9:11** *But when the multitudes knew it, they followed Him; and He received them and spoke to them about the kingdom of God, and healed those who had need of healing.*

Now ponder these questions …

- Were any of those whom Jesus healed sinners?
- Did everyone whom Jesus healed have "perfect" faith?
- Did Jesus ever refuse to heal anyone?
- Did Jesus ever turn anyone away who came to Him for healing?

- Did He ever tell anyone that it was God's will for them to be sick?
- Did He ever tell anyone that their sickness would teach them a lesson?
- Did He ever tell anyone that their sickness would glorify God in some way?

Foundation Two

Jesus is a perfect reflection of His Father. He perfectly re-presented the Father by doing what His Father did and saying what His Father said. When we look at the acts of God as demonstrated through Jesus, they point us to the very heart of God.

Read John 5:19-20.

1. The Son can do nothing of Himself, but only _____ _____.

Read Colossians 1:13-15.

2. We have been delivered from _____ and transferred into _____!

3. Jesus is the _____ of the unseen God!

Read Hebrews 1:3.

4. Jesus is the sole expression of the _____.

5. He is the perfect imprint and the very image of God's _____.

Read Hebrews 13:8.

6. If Jesus healed all when He ministered in flesh and blood on this earth 2000 years ago, He still heals today! He is the same, _____, _____, and _____!

Foundation Three

What is God's perfect will? What is God's permissive will?

God's perfect will is anything that God clearly desires for us. We know that the Word of God is the perfect will of God. We have been looking to His divinely inspired Word to see the absolute truth that it is ALWAYS His will to heal! However, God's perfect will does not mean that His desire will automatically come to pass, because even though it is clearly His desire, He has given us a free will to make our own choices.

God's permissive will refers to what God permits or allows, even though he does not desire it. Much of what happens in this world is contrary to God's perfect will. God does not cause sickness, but He does allow it.

Now for the Good News! You're not just a happenstance person out there in the mess of the world anymore. Remember, you've been delivered from the power of darkness, and have been transferred into the kingdom of the Son of His love! As a child of the Most High God, you have inherited everything in His Will (the Bible)! All of God's promises are yours! They are "in the bank"! But just as money sitting in the bank will not buy you a new car unless you withdraw the funds and make the purchase, the promises in God's Word will not result in healing unless you receive them by faith! (Stay tuned … much more to come on receiving by faith in the next few weeks!)

Foundation Four

Sickness and disease are running rampant in this world. What is in the way of God's people receiving His perfect will to heal? In this section, we will explore several possible causes for sickness and disease, or reasons why some people do not receive divine healing.

Never having received salvation

Until you become reborn, you live under the control and dominion of darkness, including sickness, disease, and eternal death. With salvation, you receive the inheritance of the King, including divine healing. Yes, God can and does sometimes heal the unsaved! But as children of God, divine healing is part of our "re-birthright"! God says yes! We say amen!

Read Romans 10:8-13.

1. When do you receive salvation?

2. What is the meaning of the word "saved" in verse 9? (G4982 – *sozo*)

◦◦◦

The importance of knowing God's complete truth

In this world, satan has whitewashed God's truth. He has watered down and diluted the gospel to be only partially true … which is in fact a lie! Most Christians believe that Jesus died for forgiveness of sins and to save us from going to hell when we die. And that's very true, praise God! But there's MORE! Jesus conquered the enemy and the curse! And then He gave us dominion over the enemy! Dominion over sin! Dominion over sickness! Dominion over darkness!

Read Hosea 4:6.

3. People perish from _____ of knowledge.

4. People perish from not _____ knowledge.

5. People perish from not _____ knowledge.

◦◦◦

The fall of man and the oppression of the enemy

When Adam gave his authority over to satan, sin entered the world, and sickness came as a result of sin. Although believers, through redemption, once again have dominion over sin and the effects of sin, the enemy is a deceiver. He is a master of oppression (an unjust or cruel exercise of authority or power). He has literally tricked many believers out of their inheritance.

Read 2 Corinthians 4:3-4.

6. Satan is the god of this world and has _____ unbelievers.

Read 1 John 5:19.

Read John 17:14-16.

7. But satan is not our god! We are _____ the world, but not _____ the world! God is our God!

Read John 10:10.

8. Satan's job description:

9. Jesus' job description:

Read John 16:33.

When we are sick, the quality of our life is lessened. When we have a chronic or terminal illness, it can cause people to question God's goodness. Satan hates God. Sickness and disease help him in his war against God's goodness by weakening us so we cannot effectively build up God's kingdom.

Disobedience to the Word of God

Sin can open the door to satan's destruction in our lives. Sin is yielding to the enemy, rather than yielding to God. This causes your heart to become hardened and insensitive toward God, and can give the enemy entrance into your soul (your mind, will or emotions), and into your body. BUT, HE HAS NO ACCESS INTO YOUR SPIRIT! Your spirit is completely perfected at the moment of salvation, washed in the precious blood of Jesus. We will explore this truth extensively is sessions 7-10 of our study.

The law of sowing and reaping

Read Galatians 6:7.
This is a spiritual law according to the Word of God. We will reap the seed we are sowing. Just as a farmer reaps a corn crop when he plants a corn seed, we can reap sickness if we sow seeds of that disease through our speaking. If you speak of a heart disease that runs in your family, you are sowing seeds of heart disease into your own future.

We can also reap what we sow through our actions. For example, if we eat poorly or don't get enough sleep, our health can suffer. If we get lots of sun without using sunscreen, we take the risk of getting skin cancer.

Life or Death … you choose

Read Deuteronomy 30:19-20.

10. God sets before us life and _____, blessings and _____.

11. Who gets to choose?

I don't know!

There are times in the life of a believer, when we simply must give up our right to understand. We know, according to the Word, that Jesus perfectly reflects His Father's will. God's Word is truth. God never changes. He does not lie. Therefore, if someone we care deeply about does not receive God's perfect will of healing, it is critically important not to waver, but to continue to live in a position of trust, even if you don't understand why that person didn't receive healing. Don't base your theology on experience. Base it on the Word of God! Base it on Jesus' life, the Word made flesh!

Trust in the Lord with all your heart, and lean not on your own understanding (or lack of understanding)!

Proverbs 3:5
(words in parentheses added by the author)

KEEPING GOD'S WORD
Receiving It, Loving It, Living It

1. Spend time daily in the Word, reading and meditating on gospel accounts of the healing miracles of Jesus. Use the lists provided in Foundation One of this session.

2. Do you know anyone who has received healing? Talk to them and have them share their story with you. You can also read documented testimonies of healing on our website at www.JesusChristHealsToday.com. Every story of every miracle or sign that God has ever performed is your story too because you have become related to the God who made them happen!

3. As you come to know the nature of God through the ministry of Jesus, then and now, an expectation will rise up within you for God's healing to be manifested in your life too!

IN PURSUIT OF MORE

My Mess – My Miracle

At the onset of my fight against stage-four cancer, I was un-saved, and ignorant regarding God's perfect will for my life.

I was deeply rooted in idolatry. God says in His Word, *"You shall have no other gods before Me or besides Me"* (Exodus 20:3 AMP). My career was my god. My priorities were completely out of alignment according to God, Who says, "Seek me first" (Matthew 6:33). God was way down on my list of priorities. My career came first, then my kids, then my husband, then my home, then many more details of life, and then, near the bottom of my priority list, was God.

I was a "high-achiever", a goal-setter and a goal-attainer. I put in long hours of hard work to bring those goals to fruition, on my own strength. I was filled with pride – pride in my own achievements, pride in our financial accomplishments, pride in my children, my marriage, my house, my "happily-ever-after" life.

I had callousness surrounding my heart, corroded by sinfulness that didn't even register in my heart as sin. Offense, impatience, harshness, vile language, and viewing and reading worldly filth, violence, and sin were all part of my everyday life.

And I sowed words and actions that had the potential to reap a harvest of death. I frequently spoke about the probability of getting skin cancer because I enjoyed the sun. I used the very minimum sunscreen protection, and spent maximum time in the sun and even in tanning booths.

Needless to say, I was positioning myself for disaster!

Right now, look back at Foundation Four in this session, where we explored several possible causes for sickness and disease. You'll see that I was primed to receive the curse, blinded by satan, the god of this world!

But that wasn't the end of my story! Jesus met me right in that place where I was, with arms opened wide in unconditional love and grace! He met me in my ignorance, in my idolatry, in my pride, in my sinfulness, in my self-inflicted word-curses of death … and He rescued me! He saved me! He revealed Himself to me! He healed me! He set me free from destruction!

All that I did was turn to Him and choose Him instead of cancer. I chose His blessing instead of the enemy's curse. I chose life instead of death. I'm very special to Abba. And so are you!

The Heart of God Revealed

In Foundation Two of this session, we see through the Word that Jesus is the perfect reflection of the Father. He perfectly re-presented the Father by doing what His Father did and saying what His Father said. When we look at the acts of God as demonstrated through Jesus, they point us to the very heart of God.

Let's take a closer look at the heart of God evidenced through Jesus in the following scriptural accounts.

John 5:1-15
A Man Healed at the Pool of Bethesda

After this there was a feast of the Jews, and Jesus went up to Jerusalem. Now there is in Jerusalem by the Sheep Gate a pool, which is called in Hebrew, Bethesda, having five porches. In these lay a great multitude of sick people, blind, lame, paralyzed, waiting for the moving of the water. For an angel went down at a certain time into the pool and stirred up the water; then whoever stepped in first, after the stirring of the water, was made well of whatever disease he had. Now a certain man was there who had an infirmity thirty-eight years. When Jesus saw him lying there, and knew that he already had been in that condition a long time, He said to him, "Do you want to be made well?"

The sick man answered Him, "Sir, I have no man to put me into the pool when the water is stirred up; but while I am coming, another steps down before me."

Jesus said to him, "Rise, take up your bed and walk." And immediately the man was made well, took up his bed, and walked.

And that day was the Sabbath. The Jews therefore said to him who was cured, "It is the Sabbath; it is not lawful for you to carry your bed."

He answered them, "He who made me well said to me, 'Take up your bed and walk.'"

Then they asked him, "Who is the Man who said to you, 'Take up your bed and walk'?" But the one who was healed did not know who it was, for Jesus had withdrawn, a multitude being in that place. Afterward Jesus found him in the temple, and said to him, "See, you have been made well. Sin no more, lest a worse thing come upon you."

The man departed and told the Jews that it was Jesus who had made him well.

This man had had an infirmity for 38 years. An infirmity is a weakness of the body or of the soul. He wasn't able to get to the pool on his own. He wasn't able to walk. And he didn't even know about Jesus and His reputation for healing, for when Jesus asked him if he wanted to be made well, he didn't immediately say, YES!!! Rather, he explained to Jesus why he couldn't get into the pool.

This man had no faith in Jesus! How could he? He didn't even know him! But what did Jesus do? He simply spoke a few simple words, and immediately the man was healed!

It's interesting that when the Jews questioned the man about the "lawfulness" of him carrying his bed on the Sabbath, he couldn't even point Jesus out to those questioning him. But Jesus made it a point to find him, and told him to sin no more, lest a worst thing come upon him.

Friends, this man was a sinner, just like I was! Jesus healed him anyway! And then Jesus gave the man direction on keeping his healing! Perhaps the reason Jesus spoke these words was to show us that the Father's heart is to heal, and that we don't need to be in a state of perfection to receive from Him!

Matthew 15:21-28
A Gentile Shows Her Faith

> *Then Jesus went out from there and departed to the region of Tyre and Sidon. And behold, a woman of Canaan came from that region and cried out to Him, saying, "Have mercy on me, O Lord, Son of David! My daughter is severely demon-possessed."*
>
> *But He answered her not a word.*
>
> *And His disciples came and urged Him, saying, "Send her away, for she cries out after us."*
>
> *But He answered and said, "I was not sent except to the lost sheep of the house of Israel."*
>
> *Then she came and worshiped Him, saying, "Lord, help me!"*
>
> *But He answered and said, "It is not good to take the children's bread and throw it to the little dogs."*
>
> *And she said, "Yes, Lord, yet even the little dogs eat the crumbs which fall from their masters' table."*
>
> *Then Jesus answered and said to her, "O woman, great is your faith! Let it be to you as you desire." And her daughter was healed from that very hour.*

The woman in this account was a Gentile. The term "Gentile" was used by Jewish people to refer to anyone who was not a member of the Jewish race. The Jews were the chosen people of God who had entered into a covenant with Him. Separation between Jews and Gentiles was very strict according to the Jewish culture of Jesus' day.

When the woman cried out to Jesus for mercy, the disciples urged Him to send the woman away. But He didn't! He talked to her about the covenant of God with Israel, and seemed to say no to her request at first. But although she wasn't a covenant person according to the Jewish culture, she worshipped Jesus. She was persistent in her seeking. Jesus recognized her great faith, and healed her daughter!

Interestingly, the definition of mercy is "where we don't get what we really deserve". The definition of grace is "where we get what we really don't deserve". The Gentile woman cried out to Jesus for mercy, but He gave her grace. She got an amazing gift that she didn't deserve, according to the Old Covenant. Jesus gave it to her anyway. Wow!

Today, as children of God, we live under the New Covenant of grace! The death of Jesus was the perfect sacrifice for the salvation of ALL, (Romans 10:12-13) and it's the will of God for NONE to perish! (2 Peter 3:9) In this account, Jesus revealed the heart of God to heal all even before the sacrifice which redeemed all was offered through Jesus, the Lamb of God!

Matthew 8:5-13
Jesus Heals a Centurion's Servant

Now when Jesus had entered Capernaum, a centurion came to Him, pleading with Him, saying, "Lord, my servant is lying at home paralyzed, dreadfully tormented."

And Jesus said to him, "I will come and heal him."

The centurion answered and said, "Lord, I am not worthy that You should come under my roof. But only speak a word, and my servant will be healed. For I also am a man under authority, having soldiers under me. And I say to this one, 'Go,' and he goes; and to another, 'Come,' and he comes; and to my servant, 'Do this,' and he does it."

When Jesus heard it, He marveled, and said to those who followed, "Assuredly, I say to you, I have not found such great faith, not even in Israel! And I say to you that many will come from east and west, and sit down with Abraham, Isaac, and Jacob in the kingdom of heaven. But the sons of the kingdom will be cast out into outer darkness. There will be weeping and gnashing of teeth." Then Jesus said to the centurion, "Go your way; and as you have believed, so let it be done for you." And his servant was healed that same hour.

A centurion was an officer in the Roman army, commanding at least 100 soldiers under him. The Roman army was considered the enemy of the nation of Israel. This centurion must have known about Jesus, and the healing that was taking place through Him. And he went outside of his "position" to seek Jesus the Healer. Notice that the moment the centurion told Jesus about his "paralyzed, dreadfully tormented" servant, Jesus said, "I will come and heal him".

But the centurion recognized that he was not worthy, because in his position of centurion he was considered Jesus' enemy, so He wouldn't allow Jesus to come under his roof. However, he expressed his faith in the authority and power of Jesus to heal.

At this point, Jesus not only recognized the man's great faith, He also compared the lack of faith of the chosen people of Israel to this soldier's faith, and painted a picture of what would result from lack of faith. The heart of God is revealed through Jesus. He is pleased by our faith (Hebrews 11:6)!

The centurion, the enemy of Israel, believed, and his servant was healed.

There is only one qualifier for receiving salvation with all of its benefits, and that is to simply believe in Jesus! The "unworthy" are made worthy when they only believe!

The heart and nature of God is revealed through Jesus the Healer. Jesus healed all who were in need while He ministered on this earth. And He still heals today. The heart of God was revealed to me when He healed me … even though I had pretty much broken every rule in His book!

Jesus is perfect theology! (Theology is the study of God and God's relation to the world.) Don't base your theology on what you see in the world. Base your theology on what you see in the Word! Healing IS God's perfect will for you!

FAITH...
SIMPLY BELIEVE

Now faith is the substance of things hoped for, the evidence of things not seen.

Hebrews 11:1

SESSION 3

> **SESSION PURPOSE**
>
> In the first two sessions of our study, we laid the biblical foundation of truth regarding God's perfect will to heal, accomplished through Jesus' death and resurrection. God has finished His part in providing for the fullness of our salvation, once and for all! Today we begin to learn about our part in receiving ALL that has been purchased for us – which is to simply believe! We will look at Abraham's example, our father in faith. And we'll explore God's way to simply believe with child-like faith!

Foundation One

Faith is our part in receiving the amazing grace gift of God, provided through Jesus' redemptive work on the cross. Let's begin our study of Bible faith by looking at God's definition.

Read Hebrews 11:1.

> Now *faith is the substance of things hoped for,* the evidence of things not seen.

What is the deeper meaning of the following words?

1. Faith –

2. Substance –

3. Hope –

Faith is the fruit of an encounter with God – the Faith-Full One! As you encounter Him, you will come to know His love, His character, His faithfulness, and His desire for you. Your faith will rise up and you will be able to say, "I am expecting something good, because I am persuaded of something true!" We will delve deep into just how we can encounter God in Session 6, "Seek the Healer".

> Now faith is the substance of things hoped for, *the evidence of things not seen.*

4. Evidence –

5. Things not seen –

In this world, we tend to believe our senses. We believe what we see, what we hear, what we feel. It does not take faith to believe what is already clearly known through our senses! But God says that faith is believing what we do NOT yet see. Faith is believing God's promises with absolute conviction BEFORE we see the manifestation!

Foundation Two

The Bible calls Abraham our father in faith. Let's look at the biblical account of Abraham to see how he stood in faith, and took action to walk by faith, not by sight.

Read Hebrews 11:8-12.

1. How did Abraham act in faith?

2. Did he understand God's plan and how it would be accomplished?

3. What did Sarah think of God's promise?

4. What was the result of their faith?

Read Romans 4:18-21.

5. What did Abraham do when then the situation was utterly hopeless?

6. Did Abraham and Sarah have reason to doubt God's promise?

7. How was his faith strengthened?

8. Why did he NOT doubt God?

Is your situation utterly hopeless according to the doctor? Does the resolution of your problem appear to be completely out of the realm of possibility? I encourage you to stand firm in faith and say, "No unbelief or distrust will make me waver concerning the promise of God, but I will grow strong and be empowered by faith as I give praise and glory to God, fully satisfied and assured that God is able and mighty to keep His word and to do what He has promised!"

Foundation Three
Child-like Faith

Where are you right now in your faith journey?
- Are you at the very beginning; just learning about God's will to heal and His good plan for you?
- Are you researching all of your options … natural, medical, and spiritual?
- Are you a "giant" of faith? Do you have a strong heart and head knowledge of the character and perfect will of God?
- Or are you somewhere in the midst of one of these entry points?

No matter where your entry point into this phase of your faith journey, Jesus tells us to become like a little child again!

Read Matthew 18:1-4. (The Message)
At about that time, the disciples came to Jesus asking, "Who gets the highest rank in God's kingdom?

For an answer Jesus called over a child, whom he stood in the middle of the room, and said, "I'm telling you, once and for all, that unless you return to square one and start over like children, you're not going to get a look at the kingdom, let alone get in. Whoever becomes simple and elemental again, like this child, will rank high in God's kingdom."

What are characteristics of childlikeness? What does it look like to be simple and elemental in our faith?

Child-like faith includes humility. Children innately know and desire to be under the authority of their parents, and they are submissive to that authority. Parents are in control! Children are absolutely dependent upon their parents.

One of the best ways to recognize God's truth is to contrast it with satan's deceptive lie. The enemy has certainly conned most of mankind into buying the massive lie that independence and being in complete control of your own life and future are powerful personal attributes. But ponder this …

1. The opposite of being humble is being full of _____.

2. The opposite of being in submission to God is being in _____ yourself.

3. The opposite of being dependent upon God is being _____.

The first step we take in nurturing humility is surrendering all to God by giving Him Lordship over every facet of our life! When we take this step of surrender, we are acknowledging our need for Him, becoming dependent on Him, and giving Him control over our lives. Surrender is the first step, and a continuing requirement of child-like faith.

Think of this analogy: A master carpenter has the ability to create a masterpiece with his hands and his tools. But if the carpenter's tools are in the workshop, not being used, they are totally useless. No work is being completed. Likewise, in order for God to create a masterpiece with our lives, we need to put our lives in His hands. We need to surrender ourselves into His care.

Read James 4:7, 10.

4. First, _____ to God. THEN _____ the devil, and he will flee!

Read 1 Peter 5:6-9.

5. It is _____ to give up control, cast your cares on God, and simply trust Him!

Word of Caution! Have you heard yourself saying, "I already know this. I don't need to learn about God's promises of healing and the prayer of faith, because I already know all about it." If so, turn back to Abba and ask Him to open the eyes of your heart to His truth, to help you to become simple and elemental again, and to deepen your revelation of His Word and His good plan for you!

> Self-Reflection: Take a minute to think about your life (your health, your relationships, your children, your career, your hobbies). Are you in control, or have you given Jesus Lordship over every area of your life? Are you dependent on God and His leading and guiding? Do you have pride in your achievements? Or have you acknowledged God as your source, and given Him the glory for blessing you with talent and ability to achieve your goals? Are you teachable?

> **Child-like faith includes trust.** Children totally trust their parents to take care of them, to protect them, to help them, to meet all of their needs.

"Trust is the fruit of a relationship in which you know you are loved."[1]

Children trust their parents because they have experienced their tender loving care, provision, and protection.

In the same way, the birthplace of trusting God is coming to know His love personally, through experience for yourself. The result of that trust is confidence, assurance, security, and dependence on God and His Word.

Read Proverbs 3:5.

6. What does it mean to "lean on your own understanding"?

> Self-Reflection: Have you completely and continuously put your trust in the Lord for your healing? Or are you striving to research and reason your problems and decisions out all on your own? Do you feel a need to understand every detail of the illness you are fighting? Or have you given up your right to understand, and – with child-like faith – simply put your trust in God?

> **Child-like faith includes simply believing.** Children believe every word their parents speak, without questioning. (That's why Santa Claus and the Tooth Fairy are so popular with many children!)

Read Luke 18:15-17. (The Message)
> *People brought babies to Jesus, hoping he might touch them. When the disciples saw it, they shooed them off. Jesus called them back. "Let these children alone. Don't get between them and me. These children are the kingdom's pride and joy. Mark this: Unless you accept God's kingdom in the simplicity of a child, you'll never get in."*

---

[1] William Paul Young, The Shack, (Los Angeles, CA: Windblown Media, 2007), 126.

FAITH... SIMPLY BELIEVE

God's Word is the pure foundation of truth for His children. Where do you base your theology? Do you base it on your experience, (or what you see in the world), or do you base it on God's Word? Do you accept the truth of God's Word with the simplicity of a child? Intellectual understanding is different than spiritual knowing. Believing does not require absolute understanding.

Read 2 Timothy 3:16-17.

7. All scripture is given by _____ of God.

Read Hebrews 4:12.

8. The Word of God is _____ and _____.

Faith begins where the will of God is known. The Word of God IS the will of God! Unless you believe with all your heart in God's completed work of healing, you will not be able to put your trust in Him to heal you!

> Self-Reflection: God expects us to believe His Word, spoken to us through the Bible. Do you question the validity of the Bible? Do you believe the words of man over the Word of God? Remember Abraham, the father of faith. He was fully convinced that what God had promised He was also able to perform. Are you fully convinced?

Child-like faith includes obedience. Children obey their parents out of trust and respect. God expects us to obey His Word, out of a deep reverence for Him and a trust that He loves us and knows best what we need.

When children trust, believe and obey their parents, the result is almost always a good, successful, happy childhood. But when children haven't been able to trust or believe their parents they very often rebel, and the result is devastating to their lives!

Read John 10:10. (NLT)
The thief's purpose is to steal and kill and destroy. My purpose is to give them a rich and satisfying life.

Yielding to the thief results in the thief's purpose coming to fruition.

Yielding to God results in God's purpose coming to fruition!

> Self-Reflection: Faith in God accompanied by obedience to His voice (His Word) will move mountains, but they must go hand in hand. Are you yielding to the enemy's lies, or to God's truth? Listen to and obey God's direction for you, whatever that is.

Child-like faith includes joy. Children are carefree, and are filled with joy and anticipation of every wonderful event in their lives!

Think about the "anticipation factor" in children. What do they do the month, the week, the day before their birthday, or Christmas, or a trip to Disneyworld? They are bubbling over, CRAZY with joy and anticipation! And they drive their parents crazy too! God wants us to be just like that as we wait upon His promises!

This characteristic of child-like faith leads us right back to the beginning of this lesson.

Hebrews 11:1a
Now faith is the substance of things hoped for ...

Here's my translation of this scripture:
I have confident and joyous expectation for God's best in my life (including healing), because I'm fully persuaded of His truth. I'm fully persuaded of His truth because I <u>know</u> Him – His faithfulness, His goodness, His amazing compassion, and His love!!!

Philippians 4:4, 6-7 (The Message)
Celebrate God all day, every day. I mean, revel in Him!

Don't fret or worry. Instead of worrying, pray. Let petitions and praises shape your worries into prayers, letting God know your concerns. Before you know it, a sense of God's wholeness, everything coming together for good, will come and settle you down. It's wonderful what happens when Christ displaces worry at the center of your life.

KEEPING GOD'S WORD
Receiving It, Loving It, Living It

1. Identify your faith "entry point" in your healing journey.
   - Are you at the very beginning; just learning about God's will to heal and His good plan for you?
   - Are you researching all of your options … natural, medical, and spiritual?
   - Are you a "giant" of faith? Do you have a strong heart and head knowledge of the character and perfect will of God?
   - Or are you somewhere in the midst of one of these entry points?

2. No matter where you enter, God's best for you is to be child-like, to go back to the beginning, to accept God's kingdom with the simplicity of a child. Take time this week to reflect on each of the attributes of child-like faith that we discussed in our study. Ask Father God to reveal His direction for you in each of these attributes. Write down your thoughts and revelations from God.

   - Humility -

   - Trust -

   - Belief -

   - Obedience -

   - Joy -

IN PURSUIT OF MORE

My Testimony of Child-like Faith

Shortly after I received my full manifestation of healing from stage-four melanoma, I asked Father God, "Show me what I did to receive my healing".

God's answer to me was so very clear. He dropped these words into my heart, "Cindy, you had child-like faith". I had no idea what child-like faith was! I didn't know what God's Word said about it. All I knew was that if I had received divine healing through my child-like faith, I wanted to learn more about it, and then share what I learned with others!

Like Abraham, there was no way in the "natural" for God's promise of healing to be fulfilled in my life.

Abraham was really old, and impotent. His wife was barren, and was long past her childbearing years. There was no way Abraham and Sarah could possibly have children, without divine intervention.

I had a stage-four melanoma diagnosis. It was considered incurable. My life prognosis was 6 to 9 months. According to the medical world, there was nothing I could do to not die within the year.

God gave Abraham a promise. He told Abraham he would be the father of many nations.

God gave me a promise. He said I would live and not die, and would declare the works of the Lord! (Psalm 118:17)

Abraham and Sarah said, "No unbelief or distrust will make me waver concerning the promise of God, but I will grow strong and be empowered by faith as I give praise and glory to God, fully satisfied and assured that God is able and mighty to keep His word and to do what He has promised!" (Romans 4:20-21)

And so did I. I chose to simply believe in my great big God, rather than the doctor's report of impending physical death. What did I have to lose?

※

This is what child-like faith looked like in me.

Within days after the stage-four diagnosis, I completely <u>surrendered</u> my health and the cancer situation to God. I had been an "in control" person all of my life, and had worked diligently to reach goals and achieve excellence in every facet of my life. For the first time ever, I simply released the problem to God, and let Him take over. I remember how freeing it was to let go of that immense burden, and give it over to the One who was able to take care of it for me! It was amazingly wonderful! Surrender was a beginning and a continuing action of faith during that season of my life (and still is!). At every turn, if the burden of sickness settled on me, I gave it over to Jesus my Healer once again!

> *Come to Me, all you who labor and are heavy laden, and I will give you rest. Take My yoke upon you and learn from Me, for I am gentle and lowly in heart, and you will find rest for your souls. For My yoke is easy and My burden is light." (Matthew 11:28-30)*

※

I immediately began to develop a relationship with Abba. My mentor told me to spend time with God every day – to read the Bible and to pray. So I did. I immediately began to experience His love for me through "God-incidences", answered prayers, and rhema words poured into my heart as I read the Bible. I began to fall in love with my Father, which caught me completely off-guard. Here I was, in the midst of a battle for my life. I started out seeking healing, and discovered the amazing love of the Healer! I came to know His compassion, His promises, and His good plan for me. My love for God was consummated as I spent time in union and communion with Him. That was the birthplace of my <u>trust</u> in God – my child-like faith.

※

As I fed on healing promises from God's Word, I chose to <u>simply believe</u> them. Believing that God had provided for my healing through Jesus was totally new to me. At that time, I didn't have biblical knowledge of the Old Testament prophecies pointing to Jesus the Healer. I didn't have biblical knowledge of Jesus fulfilling those prophecies. I didn't have biblical knowledge of the finished work of the cross, and how the power of the cross was confirmed through the book of Acts as the church was birthed. I didn't intellectually understand why healing was mine, but I chose to believe God at His Word anyway. Within one month, I began to see results in my body … proven by medical tests. And that fueled the flame of my child-like faith that it was God's will to heal me!

⋘ ⋙

I was <u>obedient.</u> I was teachable.

My spiritual mentor told me to "take the medicine" of God's healing promises daily. And I did, with all my heart.

She told me to spend time with God every day. I did, and I came to know my Healer personally.

God gave me nudges as I was reading His Word. I listened to Him. He said to ask for wisdom, and to ask in faith, knowing that He would give it to me liberally. (James 1:5) I asked Him. He gave me wisdom to ask the right questions when I got a seemingly bad PET scan report showing that the cancer was still active. God's wisdom flowed through me and enabled me to discuss the scan in depth with the technician. As a result, I walked out of that medical consultation believing that the degree of cancer was reduced. Then God confirmed the good report with His Word, "Be confident of this Cindy, that the work I have begun in you I will bring through to completion"! (Philippians 1:6)

God convicted me of unforgiveness, and set me free from demonic bondage when I obediently let go of the offense I had been harboring. He poured His blessing upon my relationship with my sister, and restored it beyond my wildest dreams! (Ephesians 3:20)

⋘ ⋙

God displaced worry and fear in my life, and it was wonderful! I lived through that season of my life with a sense of God's peace settled upon me and giving me strength. (Philippians 4:6-7, 13)

I still do. He is beyond amazing. I live in a constant state of child-likeness, depending upon Him, trusting Him, believing Him, obeying Him – in a constant state of <u>joyful anticipation</u> of what He's going to do next!

⋘ ⋙

As we continue through this healing Bible study, we will come back to many of these areas of child-like faith, and will explore biblical truth to support each of them. You will grow in revelation and deepen your understanding of the fullness of God's grace, His love for you, and His good plan for your life!

GREAT FAITH

So then faith comes by hearing, and hearing by the word of God.
                                    Romans 10:17

SESSION 4

SESSION PURPOSE

God has completed His work of healing. Jesus paid the price, once and for all, and healing became our inheritance as children of God. Our part is to simply believe! The purpose of this lesson is to reveal biblical truths about developing great faith in Jesus the Healer, to understand God's creative power over our spoken words, and to then rest in our belief that God's healing grace is more than enough!

Foundation One

Jesus teaches us the spiritual principle of praying in faith in Mark 11:22-24. The world tells us that "seeing is believing". But Jesus tells us that "believing is seeing"! Who do you choose to follow?

Read Mark 11:22-24.

1. What is a "mountain"?

2. Jesus tells us not to doubt in our _____.

3. What is our part in receiving the answer to our prayer?

4. When does Jesus tell us to believe?

5. What is the promise given to us about the prayer of faith?

6. According to Strong's Concordance, the word "receive" (G2983 - *lambano*) means _____.

7. Now read Mark 11:24 with this deeper meaning unveiled … "Therefore I say to you, whatever things you ask when you pray, believe that you _____ them, and you will have them."

Jesus teaches us to speak to the mountain. He says, "When you pray, believe that you have taken whatever you have asked of God. And you will have that for which you have prayed!"

Believing is seeing!

Foundation Two

Jesus says to have faith in God. He tells us to believe in our heart, without doubting. But how can we do that? It is a biblical truth that great faith comes through speaking and hearing God's Word.

Romans 10:17
So then, faith comes by hearing, and hearing by the <u>word</u> of God.

The Greek word for "word" in this scripture is *rhema* (G4487).
Faith comes by hearing, and hearing by the <u>rhema</u> of God.

1. Logos is the _____ Word of God.

Every word in the Bible is logos, and God inspired (2 Timothy 3:16). As we read and study the Bible, we grow in our <u>intellectual understanding</u> (logic) of His Word of truth.

2. Rhema is the _____ Word of God.

A rhema word doesn't necessarily have to be understood, only believed. Rhema is <u>spiritually knowing</u> God's Word of truth. Rhema can be deposited directly into our hearts as we read the Bible. It can be spoken into our hearts as we hear anointed teaching of the Word of God. And rhema can gradually grow in deepness within our hearts as we speak and meditate on God's promises.

Luke 1:37
For with God <u>nothing</u> will be impossible!

3. What are the 3 Greek words for the word "nothing" in this scripture?

Do you see the grave importance of God's Word revealed to your heart? When God speaks a rhema word to our inner man and we receive that word with gladness of heart, knowing that what He has spoken will come to pass, <u>great faith</u> has been birthed in us!

※※※

Read John 15:7.
The Greek word for "word" in this scripture is once again *rhema* (G4487).

    4. In John 15, Jesus tells us that He is the _____ and we are the _____.

The life of the Vine gives life to the branches. A branch does not continue to live if it is severed from the vine. But when we are vitally united to the Vine, and the Word (*rhema*) abides in us, the life of that Word is infused into us!

As His rhema word of healing is being infused into us, the life of that specific Word takes root in our hearts, and <u>great faith</u> for healing is the result! Our heart is a garden. His rhema word is the seed. And healing is the harvest!

※※※

When we pray using scriptures directly from the Word of God, we KNOW we are praying His perfect will! God's Word IS God's will!

Read 1 John 5:14-15.

    5. What is the variable in this promise?

    6. What is the guarantee in this promise?

    7. Where does our confidence come from?

As we come into agreement with God's will through speaking and meditating on his healing promises, our confidence rises up to receive His promises with gladness of heart, and that is <u>great faith!</u>

GREAT FAITH 59

Foundation Three

It is a spiritual truth that when we speak God's Word, He acts upon that Word to bring it to pass. God's spoken Word carries creative power! In the first chapter of Genesis, every time God spoke, creation took place! The worlds were framed by the spoken word of God (Hebrews 11:3).

Read Isaiah 55:10-11.

1. What is the purpose of rain and snow?

2. Compare the Word of God to the rain and the snow.

3. The Word of God shall not return _____.

4. It shall _____ that which I speak.

5. It shall _____ in the thing for which I sent it.

Read Isaiah 57:19.

6. God creates the _____ of our _____.

7. What is the meaning of the word "peace" (H7965 – *shalowm*)?

8. What is the meaning of the word "heal" (H7495 – *rapha*)?

Read Jeremiah 1:9, 12.

9. Whose words does verse 9 refer to?

10. Where are those words located?

11. What is the promise God gives us in verse 12?

In order for God's creative power to be released, His Word must be spoken. It is up to us to give voice to His Word! God is ready and waiting, actively and alertly watching and listening for His Word to be spoken, in order to perform it! Wow!

Foundation Four

God's Word is medicine!

Read Proverbs 4:4, 10, 13, 20-22.

1. Read all of these scriptures from Proverbs 4, and underline the word "live" or "life" in each scripture.

2. What is the meaning of the word "life" (H2416 – *chay*)?

3. Make a list of at least 5 directions found in these verses regarding God's Word in relation to life *(chay)*?
   1.
   2.
   3.
   4.
   5.

4. What is the result of keeping His Word in the midst of your heart?

5. What is the meaning of the word "health" (H4832 – *marpe*)?

Medical science aids healing through physical means by administering medicine into the physical body. For example, if you are fighting an infection, a medical doctor may prescribe an antibiotic for you. As you begin taking the medicine, you are confident that you will feel much better in a day or two. You don't question whether it will work. You don't worry about it. You just take the medicine as prescribed and expect it to work, and it does!

God's divine healing is spiritual. As you meditate on God's scriptural promises of healing, you are taking spiritual medicine! (Proverbs 4:22) Take the spiritual medicine of God's healing promises on a regular basis, just as you would any other medicine! Don't question whether it will work. Don't worry. It IS working … powerfully!

KEEPING GOD'S WORD
Receiving It, Loving It, Living It

Set aside time daily to meditate upon Scripture. Take this very seriously. Remember, God's word is medicine – healing and health to your flesh!

Follow these guidelines:

- Take one Scripture that God has quickened to your heart … a Scripture that speaks very closely to you or your situation; a Scripture that makes you stop your Bible reading and say, "God, what are you telling me?"

- Read it aloud several times, slowly.

- You may want to read it from several Bible translations. The website biblegateway.com is an easy place to read a Scripture from several translations.

- There may be a word within the Scripture that Holy Spirit wants to unveil to you. Look it up in a dictionary or a concordance. Strong's Concordance online is an excellent reference tool to help you study out the meaning of the biblical word in the original language. (The Old Testament was originally written in Hebrew, and the New Testament in Greek.)

- Talk to God about the Scripture. Ask Him a question if you have one. Then take quiet time to listen. Know that His voice sounds very much like your own thoughts.

- Journal your thoughts. God is speaking to you! He is revealing His heart to you.

- You may want to memorize the Scripture, or your own paraphrase of it.

- You may want to meditate on the same Scripture daily, or you may want to choose a different Scripture frequently.

IN PURSUIT OF MORE

My Testimony of Growing in Faith

The day that I accepted Jesus as my Lord and Savior, my dear friend gave me a book of healing Scriptures and told me, "This is your medicine. Pray these healing Scriptures every day." I took that little pocket book and began to read those healing Scriptures aloud day after day after day. At the beginning, they seemed like a fairy tale to me … too good to be true. I was declaring that by the stripes of Jesus I was healed (1 Peter 2:24), although the doctor's report contradicted God's report. I was declaring that the same Holy Spirit that raised Jesus from the dead was in me, and was working in my body to heal me. (Romans 8:11) But could that amazing Holy Spirit resurrection power work in me? Although I didn't understand at all … and felt totally inadequate and puny in faith, I continued to take the medicine of God's Word every day.

I began to personalize God's promises. I chose the Scriptures from the book that spoke clearly to me, and crossed out the ones that didn't. I put my own name and my own needs into those Scriptures. The fervency with which I declared God's promises grew stronger and bolder. As I continued to speak those healing declarations of God's Word aloud … something happened in my mind and in my heart. God's Word became rhema to me.

I became pregnant with the seed of God's Word. Over time, it grew bigger and stronger within my inner being. The "fairy tale" thinking gradually gave way to a spark of hope, which grew into a mustard seed of faith, which developed into a confidence in God and His promises, which gave way to excitement and joy – and great faith was birthed in my heart! I received His promises with gladness, <u>knowing</u> that His completed work of healing would come into manifestation in me. I believed and received God's report, and it trumped the doctor's report! Healed of cancer, through Jesus' redemptive work!

Meditating on God's Promises

In this world, we are really good at meditating. The problem is, we meditate on the wrong things. To meditate means to contemplate or reflect upon, to focus your thoughts upon, to ponder. The question is: what are you meditating on? Are you focusing on the problem, muddling it over in your mind, worrying about it, talking about it with countless people, and losing sleep as a result? This kind of negative meditation is the enemy's deception to divert us away from God and into fear, which is the opposite of faith!

But friends, meditation is actually God's idea! And it is a vital key in growing strong in your faith and your trust in God!

Philippians 4:8 gives us direction on what to meditate, or fix our minds on. *Finally, brethren, whatever things are true, whatever things are noble, whatever things are just, whatever things are pure, whatever things are lovely, whatever things are good report, if there is any virtue and if there is anything praiseworthy – meditate on these things.*

Meditate on God's Word in regards to healing and health and peace and strength – that's true! Meditate on your body made whole and strong – that's lovely! Meditate on the good report you are expecting – that's God's report for you too! Meditate on what you've already seen God do in your life – that's praiseworthy! Meditate on testimonies of healing – that's praiseworthy! Meditate on Jesus and how He completed the work of the cross to provide healing for you – that's really praiseworthy!

I want to give you specific guidelines on how to meditate on God's promises for healing. Remember, meditation means to reflect on God's Word, to focus upon it, to ponder it. What might that look like in action?

- Take one Scripture that God has quickened to your heart ... a Scripture that speaks very closely to you or your situation; a Scripture that makes you stop your Bible reading and say, "God, what are you telling me?"

- Read it aloud several times, slowly.

- You may want to read it from several Bible translations. The website biblegateway.com is an easy place to read a Scripture from several translations.

- There may be a word within the Scripture that Holy Spirit wants to unveil to you. Look it up in a dictionary or a concordance. Strong's Concordance online is an excellent reference tool to help you study out the meaning of the biblical word in the original language. (The Old Testament was originally written in Hebrew, and the New Testament in Greek.)

- Talk to God about the Scripture. Ask Him a question if you have one. Then take quiet time to listen. Know that His voice sounds very much like your own thoughts.

- Journal your thoughts. God is speaking to you! He is revealing His heart to you.

- You may want to memorize the Scripture, or your own paraphrase of it.

- You may want to meditate on the same Scripture daily, or you may want to choose a different Scripture frequently.

Staying Balanced

Here is the bottom line. Jesus completed the work of the cross. It is finished. Our faith does not move God to release His healing. He moved once, through sacrificing the life of His Son for our salvation, healing, and deliverance from the dominion of darkness. Faith is NOT trying to get God to heal us. Faith is believing that He already has! We access grace (God's finished work and gift for us) through faith. Faith is our choice – our choice to believe God's promises over our intellectual knowledge, our senses, our emotions, or our doctor's report.

Ephesians 2:8-9 says, *For by grace you have been <u>saved</u> through faith, and that not of yourselves; it is the gift of God, not of works lest anyone should boast.* The word "saved" in this scripture is the Greek word *sozo*, which can be more clearly translated as saved AND healed AND made well AND made whole AND delivered. Here is my paraphrase of Ephesians 2:8 … By God's grace (His free gift), through your faith (simply believing in God's finished work and gifts), you have been saved, healed, made well, made whole, and delivered!

Here is an analogy to help you to better understand the balance of grace (God's part) and faith (our part) …

Right now, there are television signals wherever you are. <u>You may not believe</u> this to be true, but your unbelief doesn't mean the signals aren't there. <u>You may not understand</u> how they work, but your lack of understanding does not mean the signals aren't there. If you plug in, turn on, and tune in a television set, you will start seeing and hearing the program. But that's not when the broadcast starts. The signal is already there. It's being broadcast 24 hours a day, 7 days a week. But you need to plug in, turn on, and tune in to receive the broadcast.

God heals today! His work is completed, and now He is "broadcasting" His healing grace 24 hours a day, 7 days a week. <u>You may not believe</u> this to be true, but your unbelief doesn't mean His healing grace isn't available. <u>You may not understand</u> God's perfect will to heal, but your lack of understanding does not halt His healing "broadcast".

Your faith is your "receiver". Unfortunately, many Christians aren't plugged in, turned on, and tuned in, and therefore their "receiver" isn't receiving! Are you connected to the Healer through relationship with Him? Are you seeking healing, or are you seeking the Healer? Do you have heart knowledge of His perfect will for you, and do you believe the truth of His will to heal? Do you know in your inner man that God is good, only good, and always good?

Another receiver problem occurs when it is out of balance. You may think that in order to receive, you must do everything just right -- pray enough, read the Bible enough, confess the word enough, never ever sin … and that THEN God is going to heal you. But this mindset says that Jesus' finished work of the cross wasn't enough, and that you need to add your works to His work in order to complete it and receive His healing grace. That mindset is not true. Faith is receiving, not achieving.

For by grace you have been saved through faith, and that not of yourselves; <u>it is the gift of God, not of works lest anyone should boast.</u> Ephesians 2:8-9

So the big question is, how do we stay in balance to receive God's grace (which includes healing) by faith? God's best for us is to simply rest in our belief that His grace is enough.

There remains therefore a rest for the people of God. For <u>he who has entered His rest has himself also ceased from his works</u> as God did from His.

Let us <u>therefore be diligent to enter that rest</u>, lest anyone fall according to the same example of disobedience. Hebrews 4:9-11

God says to enter His rest, and cease from our works. But He also says to be diligent to enter that rest! In the midst of the trial, in the midst of the questions, in the midst of the pain or suffering – rest in your belief that His grace is enough. Here's how!

Passionately and fervently enter into sweet communion with Abba. You must spend time with Him in order to grow in your relationship with Him. (John 15:4) Draw near to Him and He will draw near to you! (James 4:8) Meditate on Scriptures about God's love for you, and you will encounter His love personally. His love is the very greatest extent and the very highest degree. It is boundless. It is unfathomable. (Ephesians 3:18) And it is His greatest desire to lavish His love on you! (1 John 3:1)

Be transformed by the renewing of your mind. *Do not be conformed to this world, but be transformed by the renewing of your mind, that you may prove what is that good and acceptable and perfect will of God!* (Romans 12:2) The Greek word "transformed" in this scripture is *metamorphoo*. This is the same root word that our word metamorphosis comes from. We literally change from one form into another as our mind is renewed. The Greek word for "renewed" means a renovation, a remodel! Our old thought patterns are demolished, and completely remodeled as our mind is renewed! Meditation on God's rhema word is our primary source for renewal. Warning! Don't buy the legalistic lie that "confessing" healing scriptures over and over will get God to heal you. Rather, as you meditate on God's Word you will come to know and believe that God has already healed you, fear will be calmed and replaced with God's peace, and His Word will be established as a secure anchor for your faith.

Celebrate God's goodness. Knowing that God is absolutely good is the bedrock of your faith. Feed your heart on what God has done or is doing, not on what He does not seem to be doing. Acknowledge Him in every good thing throughout your healing journey. Journal your "God-incidences". Share your testimonies, small or large. Praise Him for His goodness in the very area in which you are seeking His grace. Exalt His name! Celebrate His goodness!

POSITIONED TO RECEIVE

Words kill, words give life; they're either poison or fruit — you choose.
Proverbs 18:21
The Message

SESSION 5

SESSION PURPOSE

The deception of the enemy is the "default operating system" of the world. Before you became a child of the King, you were under the control and dominion of darkness. But not anymore! However, the enemy is a master of deception. The purpose of this lesson is to reveal the deception of the enemy, and to reprogram your spiritual operating system to come into complete agreement with God and His good plan for you! You can move from the position of deception into the position of receiving!

The default of the world = The deception of the enemy.
As children of God, we are in the world,
but we are not of the world!

Foundation One

Meditate on God's Word. Do **not** meditate on the enemy's lies.

The default of the world (and the deception of the enemy) is to meditate on the negative. The default is to focus on the problem, to worry incessantly about it, to talk about it with countless people, to be consumed with the problem.

Read Proverbs 4:20-22.

1. Meditate means:

2. _____ is developed as you meditate on the problem.

If you are focusing your thoughts on the negative situation and constantly talking about your worries, they will be firmly established as fear within you.

3. _____ is established as you meditate on the Word of God.

As you focus your thoughts and meditate upon God's healing truths, they will become firmly established as faith in your heart.

Foundation Two

Speak words of life, **not** words of death. The power of the spoken word works in the positive and the negative. Be careful of the way you speak in everyday conversations.

The default of the world (and the deception of the enemy) is to talk about the problem, and talk about the problem, and talk about the problem. Caring people – people who love you – ask you questions about your health, which leads to more talking about the problem. What's happening in this process? You are magnifying the problem, and speaking words of death. As you magnify the problem, you are minimizing God's great plan of healing for you!

Read Proverbs 4:23-24.

1. How do you guard your heart?

Proverbs 18:21 (The Message)
Words kill, words give life; they're either poison or fruit—you choose.

Words are seeds that you sow.

2. Words of life produce the fruit of _____ and _____.

3. Words of death produce the fruit of _____ and _____.

4. Magnify _____ and His _____.

5. Don't magnify the _____!

6. As you magnify God, you _____ the problem.

Foundation Three

Receive God's truth of healing. Do **not** claim the disease you are fighting.

The default of the world (and the deception of the enemy) is to receive the bad report as <u>truth</u>. The default is to claim ownership of the disease, which is evidenced by calling it "my cancer", "my arthritis", "my Crohn's disease", etc. The diagnosis is indeed <u>factual</u>, based on medical documentation … but God's <u>truth</u> supersedes it!

1. As God's children, we don't _____ the medical report.

2. But we DO deny it's _____ to _____ in our body!

Warning:
If you agree that you <u>can</u> live with it,
you <u>will</u> live with it!

Foundation Four

Put your faith in the Healer, **not** in the doctor or the medicine.

The default of the world (and the deception of the enemy) is to put our trust and even our faith in the doctor or the remarkable treatment plan and promise. If one plan or one doctor doesn't give us our desired results, we do more research and more chasing down of the perfect miracle medicine.

Read Proverbs 3:5.

1. It's absolutely fine to seek medical help and to take medicine. But put your faith in _____.

2. _____ for your doctor.

3. _____ over your medical treatment.

Foundation Five

Read the Bible as your primary healing resource. **Be extremely cautious** of other resources and research.

The default of the world (and the deception of the enemy) is to delve into research on the diagnosis you have been given, or the treatment plan your doctor has recommended. In fact, it is seen as critical to be informed and knowledgeable about the disease and treatment protocol, including all possible side effects.

POSITIONED TO RECEIVE 71

1. God's Word brings _____ and God's _____ power.

2. Research fuels _____ and the enemy's _____ power.

Foundation Six

Keep your focus on Jesus and His completed work, **not** on your OWN works.

The default of the world (and the deception of the enemy) is to look at yourself with scrutiny in the midst of your faith journey, and question what you are doing or what you're not doing, to question your worthiness or your unworthiness, to question your strength or your weakness.

Read Hebrews 12:2.

1. Who should we be looking unto?

2. Jesus is the _____ and _____ of our faith!

3. Keep your focus on Jesus, and His finished work, not on your own works. Your faith will be _____.

4. When you focus on yourself … your works … your strength … it is a _____ to your faith.

Foundation Seven

Seek spiritual support and compassion, **not** sympathy.

The default of the world (and the deception of the enemy) is to seek sympathy, to be saturated with outpouring of love and comfort and help and support, to have others listen with pity as you share the details of the disease, treatment, pain and fear.

1. Sympathy is _____ with you in the problem.

2. Sympathy _____ the problem and it is magnified.

3. Sympathy acknowledges the problem, but cannot offer _____.

4. Sympathy offers _____ _____ rather than deliverance.

5. Sympathy is compassion's _____.

6. Compassion is _____, _____, and _____.

7. The focus and anchor of compassion is _____, and His will to heal!

Read Matthew 18:19-20.

8. What does the word "agree" mean? (G4856 – *symphoneo*)

9. You need to have others in agreement with you regarding _____, not the disease! You need others who will be _____ with you, not pity you in your weakness! You need others who will speak _____ over you, not talk with you about the problem!

One of the magnificent names of God is the great I AM. A better translation of this name for God is I AM THAT. In verse 20 of this scripture, God tells us that where two or three are gathered together in My name, there I AM THAT in the midst of them. Are you praying in agreement for God's healing to be manifest in your body? He says to you, I AM THAT in your midst! Are you praying in agreement for God's peace to guard your heart and mind? He says to you, I AM THAT in your midst! Are you praying for wisdom in making a decision? He says to you, I AM THAT in your midst!

Foundation Eight

Fill your time with the richness of God's love and truth, **not** futile, worthless time-fillers.

The default of the world, (and the deception of the enemy), is to take your mind off of your problem by filling it with worldly garbage on the television, video games, Facebook, etc.

Read Psalm 119:37.

1. Whatever you feed on the most will _____ in your life.

2. You _____ what you _____.

Foundation Nine

Seek consistency in your healing journey. **Avoid** confusion.

The default of the world (and the deception of the enemy) is overwhelming confusion during a time of tribulation. Many people with many opinions, advice, and solutions will boldly offer them to you. Spiritual options and medical options will abound … and have the potential to engulf you!

Read Psalm 71:1.

1. The anti-venom for confusion is _____ in _____.

Read 1 Corinthians 14:33.

2. God is the author of _____.

3. Who is the author of confusion?

Take an inventory of the different facets of your life: church, support groups, family, your reading and viewing. Do they all agree with God' perfect will for healing? If not, how can you resist the confusion, or better yet, remove yourself from it?

KEEPING GOD'S WORD
Receiving It, Loving It, Living It

1. What is your position in each of the nine areas we talked about in this session? Are you positioned to receive, to be deceived, or somewhere in the middle? Mark your position on each line of this chart.

POSITIONED TO RECEIVE	POSITIONED TO BE DECEIVED
Meditate on God's Word.	Do <u>not</u> meditate on the enemy's lies.
Speak words of life. Magnify your great big God!	Do <u>not</u> speak words of death. <u>Don't</u> magnify the problem!
Receive God's truth of healing.	Do <u>not</u> claim the disease you are fighting.
Put your faith in the Healer.	Do <u>not</u> put your faith in your doctor or the medicine.
Read the Bible as your primary healing resource.	<u>Be extremely cautious</u> of other resources and research.
Keep your focus on Jesus and His completed work.	Do <u>not</u> focus on your own works.
Seek spiritual support and compassion.	Do <u>not</u> seek sympathy.
Fill your time with the richness of God's love and truth.	Do <u>not</u> fill your time with futile, worthless activities.
Seek consistency in your healing journey.	<u>Avoid</u> confusion.

2. God loves you, and meets you right where you are! He will help you to move forward into His good plan for your life. Choose one area in which you would like to "reprogram" your heart and mind to believe and receive the abundant life Jesus came to purchase for us. Write it down. Tell a faith friend and ask them for their support and prayer of agreement!

IN PURSUIT OF MORE

The Waiting Room Time

One of the great difficulties during a season of fighting pain or disease of the body or soul is that of waiting on your healing. Let me start by telling you some really great news … the waiting room time is <u>a wonderful part of God's good plan for you</u>. You may not perceive it, but an immense amount of healing is happening while you wait on God … spiritual healing, emotional healing, healing of deep heart and soul wounds, as well as physical healing! In Charles Price's book, *The Real Faith for Healing*, he says, "Change externally is of necessity often superseded by change internally – transformed by His Spirit in the inner person before the manifestation of the transformation is seen in the outer person." Mr. Price goes on to say; "Often people are looking for the manifestation of God's power from the outside in, when His power only operates from the inside out."[2]

Let me share my testimony of inner healing during the six months of my life between the stage-four melanoma diagnosis, and the manifestation of God's divine healing in my body. It is with deep awe that I look back and realize how God was working so radically within me during my healing journey.

Spiritual Healing
I received the gift of salvation at the very beginning of my journey. I chose to surrender to a God I barely knew, and relinquished control of my life to Him. I received Jesus as my Savior, and gave Him Lordship over my health. Then I began developing a relationship with Abba. I started to read the Bible, and He began speaking to me through His Word! I began to spend time daily in worship and thanksgiving and prayer. God captivated my heart as I fell head over heels in love with Him. I began to meditate on His will to heal me, as evidenced through the life of Jesus Christ, and my faith blossomed.

Emotional Healing
I casted my cares upon God continuously, and I received a supernatural peace that carried me through the waiting room time. Fear was extinguished! I gave up control over every detail of my life to God, and He took over! The stress and burdens that I had grown accustomed to carrying were removed from my shoulders. Ahhhhhhhh! What an amazing relief! I reprioritized my life, and established a healthy balance for the first time ever.

---

[2]Charles Price, The Real Faith for Healing, (Gainesville, FL: Bridge Logos Publishers, 2009), 89.

Relational Healing
Several relationships in my life were radically blessed during this season.

My husband was and still is my strength, my rock. He accepted my newfound faith in Jesus. He was open to listen to my thoughts and revelations from God and His Word. My husband witnessed the new fullness of life developing within me, and made his own choice to be a Christ-follower two short months after I began my walk with Jesus.

I had a broken relationship with my sister, an offense that I had carried for over 20 years. God revealed the offense to me, I chose to let it go, and He healed my heart and restored my relationship with my sister beyond my wildest dreams!

I made a new friend during my waiting room time that changed my life forever – Jennifer, the young teacher who led me to Jesus the Healer. She was available for me, and carefully answered all of my questions with God's Word. She prayed for me. She was strong for me. She rejoiced with me!

Physical Healing
The end of God's story became the end of my story. Within six months, I was completely healed of stage-four melanoma. I had no chemotherapy or radiation. I was divinely healed, from the inside out!

The question I want to address now, is "What do I do while I'm waiting?"

First and foremost, look unto Jesus, the author and the finisher of your faith. (Hebrews 12:2) The word "look" is the Greek word *aphorao*, and it means <u>to turn the eyes and mind away from other things and fix them on something</u>. In the context of this scripture, we are to turn our eyes and attention away from all else, and fix our eyes on Jesus! As we do, our faith will rise with strength and assurance in the finished work of the cross, which has been accomplished for us!!!

Do not approach looking unto Jesus as a "work" – giving your attention to Him for a set amount of time each morning, and then getting on with your day. If you are in a "works" frame of mind, you will continuously be working to fill up your bank of faith, then use up your savings and be empty again – over and over and over. Your belief and your strength will waver, and you will be easily distracted by circumstances of life.

Instead, choose to do what Hebrews 12:2 says. Turn your eyes and mind away from all that will distract, and narrow in to a single focus … a single-mindedness … Jesus – His finished Work – His love – His joy in giving – His compassion – His will for you!

Try this. Stand up and extend both of your arms to your sides. Open your hands and hold them palm up. In one hand, visualize your body as it is today. In the other hand, visualize Jesus, and His finished work of grace. Turn your head to focus on Jesus. When you do, you can't see the distraction of your body or your problems, can you? But if you turn your head to view your body, you can't see Jesus. Danger! Danger! When you put your focus on yourself, your issues, even your own work of faith, your trust in Jesus is hindered. But when your focus is fixed upon Jesus, your faith is GREATLY strengthened!

As you fix your eyes and mind on Jesus, you will see His immense love for you, the greatest love of all, love that impelled Him to give up His very life for you. As you fix your eyes and mind on Jesus, you will see His streams of grace – salvation, forgiveness, healing, provision, abundance of life! As you fix your eyes and mind on Jesus, you will see His compassionate hand reaching out to pick you up and carry you. You will see His heart breaking for your pain ... that He's already carried for you! And you will run into His open arms and receive all that He has for you!

You will no longer say, "How can I have faith for healing? It's just too hard." Instead you will say, "I believe You Jesus. I know that you are for me, that you never leave me nor forsake me. And I trust you!" You will be at rest in faith in Jesus.

⁂

Use the time you spend in the waiting room constructively, not destructively! What are you filling your time, mind, and heart with? Often, when people are in the midst of a physical battle, they are at home with a lot of time on their hands. The tendency I've observed is that they often fill their time with the television. Contemplate this: Whatever you feed on the most will predominate in your life! Much of what is on the television and in movies is worthless, and fills your mind with idle and frequently harmful messages. Psalm 119:37 says, *Turn away my eyes from looking at worthless things, and revive me in Your way.* Follow God's advice. Turn away from the destructive choice of watching worthless things on TV.

What are constructive, healthy ways to fill your time? Set aside quality time to hang out with Abba! Talk to Him through prayer; take time to listen and journal your thoughts. Meditate on scripture. Listen to praise and worship music, and enter into heartfelt worship of the King!

Here are a few suggestions for excellent teachers to watch on television or online: Kenneth Copeland, Keith Moore, Andrew Wommack, Bill Johnson, Joseph Prince, and Joyce Meyer. These men and women of God have numerous free teachings available on I-tunes. Remember, whatever you feed on the most will predominate in your life!

༺❦༻

Don't lose heart during the waiting room time. Avoid the deception of discouragement or disappointment. It is normal for questions to arise while you are waiting. Those questions are important in your development as a believing believer. But there is danger if you allow discouragement or disappointment to lead you into deception that causes you to question the goodness of God and His will to heal.

Do not accept the lie that God isn't good, or that it may not be His will to heal you. Renounce the spirit of discouragement or disappointment!

Instead of buying the lie of the enemy, go to God and be absolutely gut level honest with Him. Talk to Him about your discouragement and your questions.

Then listen to Him. Wait for Him to respond to you. One suggestion is to read the book of Psalms until you hear your own heart's cry. Allow the balm of His Word to minister to your heart.

Receive God's peace. Important … you must give up your right to understand in order to receive the peace of God that transcends understanding. You can only hold on to one thing at a time – the promise of God, or the disappointment. You will have to drop one to embrace the other.

The goodness of God is the very bedrock of your faith. Celebrate His goodness in the very area in which discouragement is looming. Exalt the name of your Healer. Exalt the name of your Provider. Exalt the name of your Peace! Offer Him the sacrifice of your praise with all your heart. Your praise is a choice that you make, and is not based on "feeling" like praising Him!

Feed your heart on what God is doing without stumbling over what He does not seem to be doing. Leave your burden in His presence, feeding on His faithfulness![3]

---

[3] Bill Johnson, *The Essential Guide to Healing*, (Bloomington, MN: Chosen Books, 2011), 155-159.

SEEK THE HEALER

"Abide in Me, and I in you. As the branch cannot bear fruit of itself, unless it abides in the vine, neither can you, unless you abide in Me."

John 15:4

SESSION 6

SESSION PURPOSE

In Session 1 and Session 2 of *God Says Yes, We Say Amen,* we searched God's Word to come to know His will to heal. In Sessions 3, 4, and 5, we explored our part in receiving healing … which is to simply believe; to have faith in His Word. Today we come to a major juncture in our journey. The very essence of faith is the trust we have in God based on who we know Him to be through our relationship with Him. It is impossible to believe the Word of God if we don't KNOW the giver of that Word! Are you seeking healing, or are you seeking the Healer? You will not find one without the Other.

> My people are perishing from lack of knowledge.
> They don't know Me.
> They know about Me, but they don't know Me.

Foundation One

"Trust is the fruit of a relationship in which you know you are loved."[1] Saturating your mind with the truth of God's unconditional love will do more to create an environment for healing than anything else you can do. Faith to receive healing results from being open to His love.

Read Ephesians 3:17-19.

1. As you become rooted and grounded in the love of God …

2. The width of God's love …

3. The length of His love …

4. The depth of His love …

---

[1] William Paul Young, The Shack, (Los Angeles, CA: Windblown Media, 2007), 126.

5. The height of His love …

6. To know the love of God means …

Foundation Two

It is our choice, our free will, to pursue God. He's waiting with compassion and love for us to come to Him!!!

Jeremiah 29:11-13 (The Message)
> "I know what I'm doing. I have it all planned out – plans to take care of you, not abandon you, plans to give you the future you hope for. <u>When you call on me, when you come and pray to me</u>, I'll listen. <u>When you come looking for me, you'll find me.</u> Yes, <u>when you get serious about finding me, and want it more than anything else,</u> I'll make sure you won't be disappointed." God's decree.

1. What is God's plan for us?

2. What is His plan conditional upon?

Read John 15:4.

3. What does the word "abide" mean? (G3306 – *meno*)

4. What is God's condition for "fruit-bearing" in us?

Matthew 6:33 (The Message)
> *Steep yourself in God-reality, God-initiative, God-provisions. Don't worry about missing out. You'll find all your everyday human concerns will be met.*

Foundation Three
Steep yourself in the Word of God.

As we read the Word of God, we come to know the heart of the Father. We know His loving heart, and His desires for us. We know His plans for us and His promises for us. We know that He is faithful. And our faith grows.

As we read the gospels, we come to know the character of Christ. We know that Jesus was moved by compassion. We know that He fellowshipped with sinners. We know that He chose the "highly unqualified" to be His apostles. We know that He healed everyone who came to Him in need. We know that He never turned away the "unworthy". We know that He forgave unconditionally. And our faith grows.

Read Romans 12:2.
God's presence is in His Word. We become "renewed" through encounters with Him and His Word.

1. What does the word "conformed" mean? (G4964 – *syschematizo*)

2. What does the word "transformed" mean? (G3339 – *metamorphoo*)

3. What does the word "renewing" mean? (G342 – *anakainosis*)

4. What does the word "prove" mean? (G1381 – *dokimazo*)

Read 2 Timothy 3:16-17.

5. What is the meaning of the word "inspiration"? (G2315 – *theopneustos*)

6. Scripture is profitable for:

    Doctrine –

    Reproof –

    Correction –

    Instruction in righteousness –

7. The Word _____ us!

⁕

Five steps to get the most out of your time spent reading the Bible.
1. <u>Approach the Word with prayer.</u> Each day, ask God to enlighten your heart and your mind to know and understand the message He gives you through His Word.

2. <u>Read the Word slowly and carefully.</u> Read the Bible aloud, allowing the Word of God to enter your ears, your mind, and move into your heart.

3. <u>Meditate on the Word.</u> When a Scripture or passage speaks to you personally, spend time with that Scripture or passage. Reread it, recite it, say it in your own words. You may want to read the Scripture in other translations, or use a concordance to study the original Hebrew or Greek words. How does it apply to your life? Pray about it. (www.biblegateway.com is a great website to read Scriptures from different translations, and www.eliyah.com/lexicon.html is a Strong's Concordance on the web.)

4. <u>Journal your thoughts and revelations from God.</u> God is speaking to you! He is revealing His heart to you!

5. <u>Put God's Word into action.</u> When God gives you a direction or correction, take heed and make the choice to take the action or make the change God has revealed to you through His Word!

Foundation Four
Steep yourself in prayer.

Prayer is communing with God! Prayer is the turning of the human soul to the living God! Prayer is the greatest power in the world! Did you know that Jesus Himself prayed to His Father continuously? Jesus got up before dawn to pray. Jesus found time and privacy to talk to His Father constantly!

Read Mark 1:35.

1. When and where did Jesus pray?

2. What happened before this prayer time?

3. What did Jesus do right after His prayer time?

Read Philippians 4:6-7.

4. Do not _____.

5. Pray about _____ thing and _____ thing.

6. Give _____.

7. We get His _____ that will _____ our heart and mind.

Read Hebrews 4:16.

8. Why can we come boldly and confidently before the very throne of grace in prayer?

9. When we pray in our time of need, we obtain God's _____ and find His _____.

10. What is the meaning of the word "mercy"? (G1656 – *eleos*)

11. What is the meaning of the word "grace"? (G5485 – *charis*)

Foundation Five
Steep yourself in praise and thanksgiving!

As we make the choice to praise God, we enter into the presence of the Lord. He inhabits the praises of His people and strengthens us in faith as we praise! Praise changes the atmosphere. It is a dynamic, powerful force that defeats the enemy.

Read Romans 4:20-21.

1. Abraham did NOT _____ at the promise of God through unbelief.

2. Rather, he was _____ in faith as he gave praise and glory to God!

3. What was Abraham fully convinced of?

Read Psalm 34:1-4.

4. Praise God _____.

5. What is the meaning of the word "magnify"? (H-1431 – *gadal*)

6. What is the meaning of the word "exalt"? (H-7311 – *ruwm*)

7. What is the result when we praise God?

Read Psalm 103:1-5.

Make the choice to praise God and declare His goodness and faithfulness in the midst of your trial, even before you have your answer!

8. Forget not all His _____!

Read Hebrews 13:15.

9. A sacrifice involves giving God your _____, no matter what the circumstances.

10. A sacrifice of praise _____ you something! (your time, your focus, your comfort)

11. Praise is an act of your _____. Do not allow your _____ to dictate your decision to praise.

12. Praising in the midst of the battle requires _____.

It requires faith to acknowledge that His goodness and faithfulness are more real than your present difficulty. You don't need to <u>feel</u> full of faith to praise God – you just need to choose to praise Him!

KEEPING GOD'S WORD
Receiving It, Loving It, Living It

Make the choice to seek the Healer! Pursue Him!

1. Set aside a time to spend quality time alone with your Father on a daily basis. Read a chapter from the Bible. Spend a few minutes in prayer.

2. Keep a journal. Listen to your Father as you read His Word and talk to Him in prayer. Write down your thoughts and revelations. You are hearing God's voice!

3. Make the choice to praise God daily. Choose your favorite verses from the book of Psalms to praise Him with. Listen to a praise or worship CD or Christian radio. Download Christian music onto your I-pod. Watch You-Tube praise or worship videos.

IN PURSUIT OF MORE

Knowledge … Expectation … Manifestation

I want to go back to Foundation One in this session to delve a little deeper into a concept that is the absolute bedrock of faith to receive … that of coming to know the love of God and the compassion of Christ through personal experience, through intimate relationship with Abba, with Jesus, and with the Holy Spirit.

One day while praying, the Holy Spirit dropped three words into my heart – knowledge, expectation, and manifestation. I began to meditate on them. This is the revelation He has released to me to share with His children.

The first word, <u>knowledge</u>, refers to coming to know, through experience for yourself, the love of the Father and the character of Christ. How do you come to a place of knowing God so intimately? It happens in much the same way in which you come to know your spouse intimately.

I have an amazing husband and a rich, fulfilling marriage. Years ago, at the onset of our relationship, we developed a good friendship. We hung out with the same group of people. We did the usual college activities together … talking about classes, watching "Mash" on television, just hanging out with common friends, etc. But when my husband got it in his mind and heart to pursue more than a friendship with me, I saw much more deeply into his character. We began to talk and talk and talk about absolutely everything. We shared our dreams and our goals and our innermost thoughts with one another. And Kent began to pour out his love to me through his actions. He treated me like I was more precious than gold. He would drive hours to see me for just a short visit and then drive hours home. He gave me his undivided attention and utmost respect. I fell deeply in love with him, as a result of his love for me!

We have been married for over 35 years at the writing of this book, and Kent's love for me has never wavered. I know that I'm the most blessed woman in the world to have him for my husband. We continue to communicate – a LOT! We continue to spend countless hours together. He is constantly beside me, providing me with his support and strength and encouragement. He still treats me like I am more precious than gold. And my love for Kent continues to grow deeper and more secure as each year passes.

That's exactly how we grow in love with God. That's exactly how we grow in our relationship with Him! When we spend time with Him, when we talk to Him through prayer, when we listen to Him through reading His Word, when we celebrate His goodness and our joy of loving Him through praise, when we are intimate with Him through worship, we develop a deeper, more secure relationship with God our Father, the most Holy of Holies!

As a relationship grows deeper and deeper, we come to know one another really well! Over the years of our marriage, I have come to know my husband's character better than he knows it himself! We often find ourselves voicing one another's thoughts before they are even spoken! I know Kent's likes and dislikes. I know how to please him and what angers him. I know how to talk to him lovingly and respectfully about concerns, in a way that allows our conversation to be fruitful and not hurtful.

The very same thing happens in our relationship with our Father! As our relationship with God grows deeper and deeper, we come to know Him really well! As we read the Word of God, we come to know who He is. We know what blesses Him and what hurts Him. We know His loving heart, and His desires for us. We know His plans for us. We know His promises for us, and we know that He is faithful!

As we read the gospels, we come to know the character of Christ. We know that Jesus was moved by compassion. We know that He fellowshipped with sinners. We know that He chose the "highly unqualified" to be His apostles. We know that He healed everyone who came to Him in need. We know that He never turned away the "unworthy". We know that He forgave unconditionally.

I love the words Jesus spoke to the Father about you and me, in the 17th chapter of John. He said: *I have made Your Name known to them and revealed Your character and Your very Self, and I will continue to make [You} known, that the love which You have bestowed upon Me may be in them [felt in their hearts] and that I [Myself] may be in them.* (John 17:26 AMP)

My friend, consistently, diligently seek the Healer. Express your hunger and your desire to know Him personally. And you will find Him. You will come to know Him intimately, and to receive His amazing love!

≈≈≈

The second word God dropped in my heart was the word <u>expectation</u>. Let me go back to my relationship with my husband in order to reveal God's heart to you. Over the years, I have come to have certain expectations of my husband, simply because he has proven to me through his consistent character that he is who he is. For example, I expect to hear him tell me how much he loves me and how beautiful I am multiple times every day. He's done that for over 35 years, and I expect him to continue! I expect a cup of coffee to appear every morning as I am putting on makeup and doing my hair. He's done that for years, and I wait in expectation daily for my coffee to arrive. And it does! On a more serious note, I completely trust my husband. He has displayed his unconditional love for me consistently over all these years. And "trust is the fruit of a relationship in which you know you are loved!"[1]

This same kind of expectation results as we come to know the love of the Father and the character of Christ, and to see that love and character evidenced through experience.

I started spending time with God daily the very first day I was saved, and that time has grown richer and richer over the years. As I've grown in my relationship with God, I've experienced His promises coming to pass in my life! It began with little things, like unexpected favor and "God-incidences" happening way too often to be coincidences. Then I began to see things in my body change in accordance with God's promises. Within six months after the initial diagnosis of stage-four incurable melanoma, I was declared cancer free, with no medical treatment. But it didn't end there! Within a few months, I shared my story with three other people who were also fighting the war against cancer. One man had terminal brain cancer. Another had been diagnosed with high-grade sarcoma. And the third was a dear friend whose son was being tested for leukemia. All three diagnoses were reversed within a very short time, with the doctors simply not understanding why! At that point, I was completely overwhelmed with an awe of God and His promises and His faithfulness!

Since then, through my years of growing in the ministry of healing – I have been feeding on God's Word about healing constantly, explaining it and proclaiming it every chance I get. Now when we hear of the miraculous outcomes of the people we are ministering to, I'm not even surprised. Why? Because I EXPECT them to receive healing! I KNOW Jesus is the Healer! I KNOW that it is God's perfect will to heal. I KNOW that when the people have knowledge, and receive it into their hearts, their faith connects to the Power Source, and healing results!

Expectation comes as a result of knowing God through experience for yourself! "Trust is the fruit of a relationship in which you know you are loved!"[1] Trusting God is the foundation of faith. Heart faith opens heaven's windows for us to receive!

The third word, of course, is <u>manifestation</u>. Manifestation is the result of expectation, which is the result of personally knowing God's love and the character of Christ. Manifestation is healing and continued health, and so much more! Manifestation is God's tender love displayed before your eyes. Manifestation is being completed because Jesus lives within you. Manifestation is a deep desire birthed in you to read the Bible, because you are so ravenous for the manna of God's Word. Manifestation is an energy that surges through you as you talk about God's promises and His plan for you. Manifestation is a hurting heart that has been healed or a relationship that has been restored.

[1] William Paul Young, The Shack, (Los Angeles, CA: Windblown Media, 2007), 126.

You see, when you seek the Healer, the result is so much more than just healing!

❧❧❧

You are responsible for your love relationship with God!

How many marriages don't end up like Kent's and mine? How many marriages fall apart, with the man and woman falling out of love instead of deeper into love? The same thing can happen with God Almighty … not because of God, but because of us. God is love. And the Love that is God is deeper and wider and higher than we can possibly perceive.

But a relationship involves two parties. If we don't continue to seek God, our relationship with Him will falter and wither up. God reveals this truth in His Word. *I am the Vine; you are the branches. Whoever lives in Me and I in him bears much (abundant) fruit. However, apart from Me [cut off from vital union with Me] you can do nothing. If a person does not dwell in Me, he is thrown out like a [broken-off] branch, and withers; such branches are gathered up and thrown into the fire, and they are burned.* (John 15:5-6 AMP)

Purpose in your heart to seek His face, to require Him as a vital necessity, to <u>know</u> Him intimately, to <u>expect</u> His loving response to you, and to receive His <u>manifest</u> glory!

Knowledge … Expectation … Manifestation!

Living in the Fullness of the Holy Spirit

I have talked a lot about knowing Abba your Father, and knowing Jesus your Healer, but there is more … LOTS more! The <u>source</u> of healing is the Father, the giver of every good and perfect gift. The <u>deliverer</u> of that gift is Jesus. And the <u>power</u> of the source is the Holy Spirit.

When Jesus was walking on this earth in the form of a man, He promised us another Helper. In John 14:16-17 Jesus says, *"And I will pray the Father, and He will give you another Helper, that He may abide with you forever – the Spirit of truth, whom the world cannot receive, because it neither sees Him nor knows Him; but you know Him, for He dwells with you and <u>will be in you</u>."*

Jesus was referring to the outpouring of the Holy Spirit's baptism upon believers after His ascension into heaven, which is available for you today.

There are two HUGE benefits that come with the infilling of the Holy Spirit. The first benefit is to have the fullness of the power of the Holy Spirit at work <u>within you</u> for the purpose of developing and becoming strengthened spiritually. The Holy Spirit will teach you all things, and

He will bring to your remembrance what Jesus has already spoken to you. (John 14:26) The Holy Spirit will reveal the deep things, or mysteries, of God to you. (1 Corinthians 2:10-12, 14:2) The Holy Spirit within you builds you up spiritually, and energizes your faith. (1 Corinthians 14:4; Jude 1:20)

But there's even more! In Acts 1, *Jesus commanded His disciples not to depart from Jerusalem, but to wait for the Promise of the Father, "which," He said, "you have heard from Me; for John truly baptized with water, but you shall be baptized with the Holy Spirit not many days from now."* (vs. 4-5) And He said to them, *"But you shall receive power <u>when the Holy Spirit has come upon you</u>; and you shall be witnesses to Me in Jerusalem, and in all Judea and Samaria, and to the end of the earth."* (vs.8)

The second benefit of the Holy Spirit baptism is to have the fullness of the power of the Holy Spirit at work <u>upon you</u> to witness, to preach, to heal, to deliver. (Acts 1:8; Mark 16:15-18)

We were created to be "Power-assisted". Think of the power steering on an automobile. If you've ever had your power steering go out on your car, you know that you can still steer, but it is incredibly difficult! However, with the benefit of power steering, you can steer effortlessly. In much the same way, we can function without the Holy Spirit baptism. We are still in communion with God. We are still in a position of rightstanding with Him. We are still a receiver of His blessings and inheritance. But we don't have the added benefit of being "Power-assisted"!

Let me define the biblical word "power" that is in Acts 1:8 … *But you shall receive <u>power</u> when the Holy Spirit has come upon you …*

The Greek word for this word is *dynamis*. It is the root word that our English word dynamite comes from. *Dynamis* is inherent power, residing in a Holy Spirit filled believer by virtue of the Holy Spirit's nature within and upon him. Dynamis is miracle-working power. Dynamis is power such as that which rests in armies, forces, or hosts (like angel armies!!!!).

I know that my own baptism in the Holy Spirit impacted my lifelong healing journey more than anything else except receiving my salvation. I believe that the very reason that I had great faith to receive my own healing of stage-four cancer was because of the fullness of the Holy Spirit within and upon me. I believe that the very reason that I am anointed to preach and publish God's truth today is because of the fullness of the Holy Spirit within me. I believe that the very reason that I am anointed to lay hands on the sick and witness signs and wonders and healings is because of the fullness of the Holy Spirit upon me.

The big question is "How do you receive this amazing Promise"? The answer is simple. Just ask! Many have not because they ask not! (James 4:2) Jesus told us in Luke 11:13, *"If you then, being evil, know how to give good gifts to your children, how much more will your heavenly Father give the Holy Spirit to those who ask Him!"*

So ask Father God. Simply ask Him with your own words, expressing your desire for the infilling of the Holy Spirit. Or use this prayer, and ask God from the depth of your heart …

Father, Your Word says that the Holy Spirit is a gift. I do not have to work for it. All I need to do is ask and receive it. So I ask You to baptize me now with Your Holy Spirit. I desire Your impartation in every part of my life. I want to receive all that You have for me! My heart cry is for a radical transformation in my walk with You. Consume me, O God, with Your holy fire! I receive right now, Your Promise, Your Gift, the Baptism of the Holy Spirit.

༺❀༻

The biblical evidence of the baptism of the Holy Spirit is that of speaking in tongues. We see this in the book of Acts as the outpouring of the Holy Spirit came upon hundreds and hundreds of believers. (Acts 2:1-4; Acts 10:44-46; Acts 19:1-7) The epistles repeatedly refer to speaking in tongues and praying in the spirit. (Romans 8:26-27; 1 Corinthians 2:13; 1 Corinthians 14; Jude 1:20) Yes, the promise of the Holy Spirit is for you today! (Acts 2:38-39)

The benefits of the Holy Spirit within you for spiritual growth and revelation, and upon you for power – are activated as you pray in tongues. I pray in tongues daily. I am built up in the Holy Spirit, I am led by the Holy Spirit, I am empowered by the Holy Spirit as I pray in tongues. I have a relationship with the Father, the Son, and the Holy Spirit … and it's beyond amazing!

GODLY LIVING

But as he who called you is holy, you also be holy in all your conduct, because it is written, "Be holy, for I am holy."

1 Peter 1:15–16

SESSION 7

SESSION PURPOSE

God has an amazing plan for your life. Jesus tells us, *"The thief's purpose is to steal and kill and destroy. My purpose is to give them a rich and satisfying life."* (John 10:10 NLT) In this teaching, we look at how to receive Jesus' purpose and reject the thief's purpose! Don't give the enemy a foothold. Yield to God, not to the enemy!

Know His will.
Pray His will.
Yield to His will.

Foundation One

As born again children of God, we have been made righteous, and we no longer live under the dominion (control) of sin.

Read Romans 6:5-7, 10-14.

As born again believers, we share in the death of Jesus.

1. Our old man was _____ with Jesus, so that we should no longer be _____ of sin.

2. For one who dies is _____ from sin.

As born again believers, we also share in the resurrection of Jesus! For by the death He died, He died to sin once and for all, and then He was resurrected to new life in unbroken fellowship with God.

3. We too now live in _____ _____ with God, because of the sacrifice of our Savior!

4. Why doesn't sin have dominion (control) over us any more?

Romans 8:2-3 (AMP)

For the law of the Spirit of life [which is] in Christ Jesus [the law of our new being] has freed me from the law of sin and of death.

For God has done what the Law could not do, [its power] being weakened by the flesh [the entire nature of man without the Holy Spirit]. Sending His own Son in the guise of sinful flesh and as an offering for sin, [God] condemned sin in the flesh [subdued, overcame, deprived it of its power over all who accept that sacrifice],

5. Sin is deprived of its _____ over all who accept Jesus' sacrifice.

When we surrendered our hearts to Jesus, declared our belief in Him, and gave Him Lordship over our lives, we accepted the sacrifice of Jesus and reaped the benefits of grace.

6. At that very moment, our born-again spirit was created in a state of _____.

Foundation Two

Righteousness is not synonymous with holiness. Righteousness is a gift. Holiness is a choice.

Read 2 Corinthians 5:21.

Righteousness clarified (G1343 – *dikaiosyne*; as defined in Vines Expository Dictionary of New Testament Words)

1. Righteousness is the gracious _____ of God whereby all who _____ in the Lord Jesus Christ are brought into right relationship with God.

2. It is unattainable by our _____ to any law, or our own _____, or our _____.

3. Righteousness is based entirely upon receiving what _____ has done.

4. It is not something we _____. It is something we _____.

5. Our _____ is perfected in this state of righteousness.

Read 1 Peter 1:14-16.

Holiness clarified (G40 – *hagios*; as defined in Vines Expository Dictionary of New Testament Words)

6. Our _____ and _____ are not made perfect at the time of salvation.

7. Holiness is not a gift from God, but a decision of _____ in man by his own free will.

8. God supplies the _____, man supplies the submission and obedience to the Word of God, and _____ is the result.

9. Holiness is something we _____. It is a _____.

Foundation Three

God has provided all that we need in order to grow in holiness all the days of our lives. Think of your heart as a garden. On the day you invited Jesus to be the Lord of your life, He entered into your heart. But that garden may still have a lot of weeds in it from your "former" life. As you sow the seed of God's Word into your heart, it grows a pervasive ground cover, completely taking over your heart, and literally choking out the weeds (the corruption, defilement, sin-tendencies) of your heart!

Read 1 Thessalonians 5:23.

1. What does the word "sanctify" mean? (G37 – *hagiazo*)

2. Do you sanctify yourself?

3. What parts of us will be preserved blameless (carefully attended and taken care of)?

Read John 17:15-17.

4. What does Jesus pray we will be sanctified through?

5. Unless we're shaped by the _____, we'll be shaped by the _____.

Read Ephesians 5:25-26.

6. The water of the Word sanctifies and cleanses us from the _____ of life.

7. The Word of God cleanses us, woos us, draws us nearer to God. The _____ you come to God, the less junk you can take with you!

2 Corinthians 3:18 (AMP)
And all of us, as with unveiled face, [because we] continued to behold [in the Word of God] as in a mirror the glory of the Lord, are constantly being transfigured into His very own image in ever increasing splendor and from one degree of glory to another; [for this comes] from the Lord [Who is] the Spirit.

8. We are transformed (sanctified) by beholding the glory of the Lord in the _____ _____.

9. We _____ what we _____.

2 Peter 1:3-4 (NLT)
By his divine power, <u>God has given us everything we need for living a godly life</u>. We have received all of this <u>by coming to know him</u>, the one who called us to himself by means of his marvelous glory and excellence. And because of his glory and excellence, he has given us great and precious promises. These are the promises that <u>enable you to share his divine nature and escape the world's corruption caused by human desires.</u>

10. Sanctification is when we let God _____.

11. This happens by _____.

Foundation Four

Remember that when we accepted Jesus' sacrifice, our born again spirit was created in a state of righteousness. When we sin, that sin does not affect our rightstanding with God. When we sin, it does not affect God's love for you.

But sin does have consequences – not on your born-again spirit. It's your soul or your body that get contaminated and defiled.

Notice the parallel between sin and sanctification.

SIN	SANCTIFICATION
Separation FROM God and UNTO the world	Separation FROM the world and UNTO God
Yielding to the enemy (worldliness)	Yielding to God (godliness)
Heart becomes hardened, cold, insensitive, unyielding and unfeeling toward God	Heart grows progressively more sensitive to sin, and open to hear God's loving voice of conviction and correction.
Opens a door to the enemy to gain access into your soul or your body	No open access to the enemy to invade your soul or your body

Ephesians 4:17-19 (NIV) -- A lifestyle of sin
So I tell you this, and insist on it in the Lord, that you must no longer live as the Gentiles do, in the futility of their thinking. They are darkened in their understanding and separated from the life of God because of the ignorance that is in them due to the hardening of their hearts. Having lost all sensitivity, they have given themselves over to sensuality so as to indulge in every kind of impurity, and they are full of greed.

Ephesians 4:22-27 (NIV) -- A lifestyle of sanctification
You were taught, with regard to your former way of life, to put off your old self, which is being corrupted by its deceitful desires; to be made new in the attitude of your minds; and to put on the new self, created to be like God in true righteousness and holiness.

Therefore each of you must put off falsehood and speak truthfully to your neighbor, for we are all members of one body. "In your anger do not sin": Do not let the sun go down while you are still angry, and do not give the devil a foothold.

Foundation Five

Under the Old Covenant, sin was atoned for. The word atonement meant that sins were covered over. The sin offering had to be repeated year after year because it only covered the Israelites' sins. Their sin nature still remained in them.

But Jesus came to pay the complete penalty for our sin, so that ALL sin -- past, present, and even future -- would be remitted. Remission of sins is a gift to all children of God who have accepted Jesus' sacrifice.

The word remission means
- We have been released from the penalty that we owed, because Jesus paid it for us.
- All the damages of our sins have been paid off, and reparation has been made.
- Sin has not just been covered or hidden; it has been eliminated! All sin has been completely removed from us. It is just as if our sins had never been committed.
- Jesus completely conquered sin.

The awesome result of the remission of our sins is that we are eternally separated from sin, and eternally reconciled to God!

Read Matthew 26:28.

1. How was the New Covenant ratified?

2. What was the result of the New Covenant?

Read Ephesians 1:7.

3. What does the word "redemption" mean?

4. The word "forgiveness" in this scripture is the exact same Greek word as the word _____.

Foundation Six

Sin does not affect God's love for us. It does not affect our righteousness. The blood sacrifice of Jesus has provided for the remission of all of our sin. But heart repentance is crucial! Why? Because God wants to do more than just get us out of the red. He wants to get us into the black! Yes, your debt is paid in full. But He wants you to readily receive His benefits!

Read Romans 2:4.

1. When we make mistakes and yield to the enemy instead of God, we need to run back into the arms of Abba in a position of _____ and _____ to His grace.

2. Repentance is the result of a truly _____ heart. It is a result of renewing your mind to God, His goodness, His forgiveness – and then _____.

3. Turning from sin to God is the result of _____.

4. In this process of surrendering to the grace of God and repentance, the enemy's access to your soul or your body is _____!

Read 1 John 3:21-24.

"If our heart does not condemn us" means …

5. We are confident in our God because we know our position of _____ in Christ.

6. We grow in _____ as we come close to Abba with a heart of surrender and yieldedness to His loving voice of conviction and encouragement.

7. We keep His Word when we _____ and _____.

8. What is God's promise for us as a result?

KEEPING GOD'S WORD
Receiving It, Loving It, Living It

1. Take a look back at yourself before you knew Christ or rededicated yourself to Him. Contrast the person you were then to the person you are now.

2. What is an area of your life in which you have grown?

3. What is one area in your life in which you want to grow? Write it down. Tell one person your desire, and ask him/her to help hold you accountable for this area of sanctification.

IN PURSUIT OF MORE

My Testimony of Growing in Godly Living

As I look back in time, it is clear that before I came to the fullness of the knowledge of Christ, and who I am in Christ, I ignorantly lived in darkness, blinded by the enemy. My soul was calloused from a lifetime of yielding to the enemy and worldliness. The area of my life that harbored the gravest sin was in the realm of my priorities. I was an in-control person, striving to accomplish my own agenda, my own plan, my own purposes and passions. I was self-righteous, and attributed my talents and accomplishments to my own hard work. I was driven to succeed in my career. I was an early education teacher who had recently been promoted to the position of Learning Consultant, a position of leadership and high esteem. My next goal was to become a building administrator, and possibly move on to district or county level administration. I worked hard and long in my own strength. My family paid the price. Although I managed to play the role of chauffeur and home manager quite effectively, my first love was my job. As far as God went, I ushered the family to church religiously every Sunday, planned my daily to-do list during the sermon, and checked God off my list for the week.

My priorities changed radically when I began seeking Jesus. He says to seek Him and you will find Him (Luke 11:9); abide in Him and He will abide in you (John 15:4); draw near to Him and He will draw near to you (James 4:8). And He is faithful to His word! I found Him, pure and simple. I fell in love with Him. He captured my heart. I gave Him my life. I continue to seek Him first every single day. My heart has become sensitive to His voice, to His presence, to His love for me. I made the choice to yield to God … and He did the rest! I made the decision NOT to pursue becoming an administrator. God had lots for me to learn and do right where I was. My purpose and my passion shifted to growing in my relationship with Abba, and to live with Him, in Him, and for Him, all the days of my life! I made the decision to purchase years of service in education so that I could retire early, and devote my time, my resources, and my gifts totally to God! Now THAT was a change of heart!

Another example of growing in godly living involved filtering what I allowed to enter my heart through my ears and my eyes. In my past, I had grown insensitive to watching or reading about lust, sex, evil, or violence. In this world, sin is not even seen as sin any longer! And I was enmeshed in the world. My favorite genre of fiction was what I called "smut novels" -- the more explicit the better. After I received Jesus as my Lord, and began seeking Him, my heart became sensitive to His heart, and I no longer wanted to read filth. I threw all of my trashy books in the trash. The same thing happened with my viewing. In my past, I could watch violence, sex, and profanity on TV or movies, with absolutely no effect on my conscience. But not after I came to know my Father. I increasingly became more and more sensitive to His heart and to His voice.

As I was in the process of writing this very lesson, my husband and I watched a movie rated PG13 that was a romantic comedy – but it had LOTS of killing in it. God spoke to me during the night after viewing that movie. He told me not to be entertained by the devil's play. He told me to guard my heart and my mind. He told me to keep myself pure, and conditioned to receive and do as directed and led by Him! I have grown sensitive to my Father and passionately desire to please Him and grow in my walk with Him!

The final example of growing in holiness that I'd like to share is that of learning to listen with kindness and compassion to others. In my job as a Learning Consultant, it was my responsibility to advocate for children, parents, and teachers on an ongoing basis. But when I didn't have time to converse at length, I would abruptly end conversations, letting the person at hand know I had important things to attend to. God convicted me of this as I came into relationship with Him. He was always there for me. He always listened to me with such compassion. He always had time for me. He always answered my questions, and guided me step by step. So I made a decision to change my behavior. I chose "active listening" as one of my personal yearlong goals as an educator. I asked two colleagues who were strong believers to be my accountability partners, and to tell me if/when they noticed me not actively and kindly listening and responding to others. And they did. Over time, I grew to more closely resemble my Father in this area of my life.

Godly living is a choice. It is a lifelong process. God supplies the grace. We supply the submission and obedience. Holiness is the result.

Consequences of Sin

In this Session, I shared the truth that your spirit is perfected the moment you accept Jesus' sacrifice. Jesus wiped out your record of sin, and He wiped out sin's power over you. But, as we learned, sin does have consequences. It does not affect your spirit EVER AGAIN, but it does have a destructive effect on your soul, which could lead to emotional wounds, physical pain or disease. We will learn more about unknowingly giving the enemy a foothold or stronghold into your soul and how to evict him in Session 9. But at this point, I would like to share a few examples of very real consequences of sin on your soul and on your physical body.

- Unforgiveness is a sin that can lead to bitterness, strife, and broken relationships. Bitterness and strife can in turn end up in physical pain and disease. Research shows that the most common root cause of disease involves psychosomatic issues. This refers to a physical disorder that is caused or greatly influenced by emotional factors.

- Worry and anxiety are literally sin (Romans 14:23, Philippians 4:6). They can lead to a buildup of stress, which is known to cause muscle pain, digestive issues, increased blood pressure and cholesterol, heart disease or strokes, compromised immune system, allergies, rheumatoid arthritis, or cancer metastasis.

- The sin of drunkenness can lead to broken relationships, broken marriages, addiction, disease, and ultimately death.

- Sexual immorality can lead to unhealthy soul ties, pornography addiction, unwanted pregnancies, and sexually transmitted diseases.

These examples are just a sampling of very real consequences of sin in your soul or your body. But God has a better way! Yield to Him and see!

The Sum Total of God's Commandments

Jesus sums up our Father's expectations for us in two statements:

> *"Teacher, which is the most important commandment in the law of Moses?"*
>
> *Jesus replied, "'You must love the Lord your God with all your heart, all your soul, and all your mind.' This is the first and greatest commandment. A second is equally important: 'Love your neighbor as yourself.' The entire law and all the demands of the prophets are based on these two commandments." (Matthew 22:36-40 NLT)*

Love God. What does that look like? We have been reconciled to God through salvation. And He desperately desires us to spend quality time with Him! Praise Him! Worship Him! Talk to Him! Listen to Him! Be intentional in seeking Him first every single day of your life.

Love others. This second commandment flows naturally out of the first. All of man's best efforts towards loving others will fail as long as we attempt to do it on our own, without God. But as we seek God, and come to know Him personally and intimately, our hearts and minds are transformed by the indwelling presence of the Holy Spirit. We are able to love others as we reflect God's ultimate expression of love. We become what we behold. Paul paints a picture of what loving others looks like in action with these words:

> *Since God chose you to be the holy people he loves, you must clothe yourselves with tenderhearted mercy, kindness, humility, gentleness, and patience. Make allowance for each other's faults, and forgive anyone who offends you. Remember, the Lord forgave you, so you must forgive others. Above all, clothe yourselves with love, which binds us all together in perfect harmony. And let the peace that comes from Christ rule in your hearts. For as members of one body you are called to live in peace. And always be thankful.*
>
> *Let the message about Christ, in all its richness, fill your lives. Teach and counsel each other with all the wisdom he gives. Sing psalms and hymns and spiritual songs to God with thankful hearts. And whatever you do or say, do it as a representative of the Lord Jesus, giving thanks through him to God the Father. (Colossians 3:12-17 NLT)*

God says to have mercy, be gentle, be patient, make allowances for others faults, and forgive those who offend you. Okay, that's not so bad when people around us "play nice". But what if they don't? What about the "unloveable" people? The ones who are not godly in any fashion whatsoever, the ones who are rude and spiteful and cantankerous?

> Jesus said, *"But I tell you, Love your enemies and pray for those who persecute you, to show that you are the children of your Father Who is in heaven; for He makes His sun rise on the wicked and on the good, and makes the rain fall upon the upright and the wrongdoers [alike].*
>
> *For if you love those who love you, what reward can you have? Do not even the tax collectors do that? And if you greet only your brethren, what more than others are you doing? Do not even the Gentiles (the heathen) do that?* (Matthew 5:44-47 AMP)

The gist of this message is that God blesses all of us, regardless of our "goodness". He pours out His sunshine and His rain on the wicked and the good. He sent Jesus, who knew no sin, to become sin for us.

> *But God demonstrates His own love toward us, in that while we were still sinners, Christ died for us.* (Romans 5:8)

Yes, it's easy to love those who love us. But God directs us to love our enemies, and to pray for them.

We are not alone in this process. We have the Holy Spirit to guide us, and the Word of God to cleanse us. (1 Peter 1:22-23) Father God assures us that His will is for us to grow mature in godliness in our mind and our character. (Matthew 5:48)

He said it. I believe it. That settles it!

FORGIVE,
AS YOU HAVE BEEN FORGIVEN

"And whenever you stand praying, if you have anything against anyone, forgive him, that your Father in heaven may also forgive you your trespasses. But if you do not forgive, neither will your Father in heaven forgive your trespasses."

Mark 11:25–26

SESSION 8

SESSION PURPOSE

The Word of God clearly speaks of the need for us to forgive … to forgive as we are forgiven, to forgive repeatedly if needed, to freely forgive others from our heart of all their offenses (Matthew 18:35). Why? Because Jesus loved us to the death in order to bring us into reconciliation with God, and separation from sin, separation from bitterness and its effects, separation from woundedness and emotional pain. Unforgiveness is a bait of satan, designed to establish bitter roots within our heart, and to provide the deceiver with a stronghold into our soul. Bad roots grow bad fruit – fruit of strife and pain and disease. God's best for us is to forgive. Don't give the devil a foothold! (Ephesians 4:27)

Foundation One

The redemption of Christ brought forgiveness. When we accept the holy sacrifice paid for by our Savior, we are set free from the bondage of sin. The record of our sin is voided. The debt we owed is canceled out. We are forever forgiven!

Read Ephesians 1:7.

1. What does the word "redemption" mean?

2. The word "forgiveness" in this scripture is the exact same Greek word as the word
   _____.

Forgiveness includes remission! Remission means that we have been released from the penalty that we owed, because Jesus paid it for us. Remission means that all sin has been completely removed from us. The awesome result of the remission of our sins is that we are eternally separated from sin, and eternally reconciled to God!

Foundation Two

We are forgiven! That's WONDERFUL news! But Jesus says we are to forgive, just as we have been forgiven. In fact, He says it over and over in the Word of God. His Word is truth, and the truth will set you free!

Matthew 6:12, 14-15
"And forgive us our debts, As we forgive our debtors.

For if you forgive men their trespasses, your heavenly Father will also forgive you. But if you do not forgive men their trespasses, neither will your Father forgive your trespasses."

Matthew 18:32-35
"Then his master, after he had called him, said to him, 'You wicked servant! I forgave you all that debt because you begged me. Should you not also have had compassion on your fellow servant, just as I had pity on you?' And his master was angry, and delivered him to the torturers until he should pay all that was due to him.

So My heavenly Father also will do to you if each of you, from his heart, does not forgive his brother his trespasses."

Mark 11:25-26
"And whenever you stand praying, if you have anything against anyone, forgive him, that your Father in heaven may also forgive you your trespasses. But if you do not forgive, neither will your Father in heaven forgive your trespasses."

Luke 6:37
"Judge not, and you shall not be judged. Condemn not, and you shall not be condemned. Forgive, and you will be forgiven."

Ephesians 4:32
And be kind to one another, tenderhearted, forgiving one another, even as God in Christ forgave you.

Colossians 3:13
bearing with one another, and forgiving one another, if anyone has a complaint against another; even as Christ forgave you, so you also must do.

The redemption of Christ freed us of all of our sin and released us from the penalty we owed. So why is God's requirement for us to forgive directly connected to receiving His forgiveness?

Unforgiveness is a hindrance to our faith. It can so occupy our heart that it leaves no room for believing. We must believe in order to receive the benefits of His grace, including forgiveness!

Foundation Three

Unforgiveness opens the door for the enemy to gain a foothold into your soul.

Matthew 6:14-15 (The Message)
> *In prayer there is a connection between what God does and what you do. You can't get forgiveness from God, for instance, without also forgiving others. If you refuse to do your part, you cut yourself off from God's part.*

Read Matthew 18:21-35.

1. Jesus uses this parable to teach about forgiveness. The servant owed the king 10,000 talents, which is equal to about $10,000,000! What did the king do when his heart was filled with compassion?

2. That same servant was owed about a hundred denarii by one of his peers, which is equal to about $20! What did he choose to do?

When we have been forgiven by God for so great a debt, yet refuse to forgive others, our spiritual cover is blown. We are unprotected. We open the door to let the "torturers" take advantage of our lack of protection. We become easy prey to the demonic realm.

One of the enemy's tactics is to lure us with the subtle bait of offense, set in a trap that has the ability to snare us in the miry pit of bitterness and unforgiveness.

Read Luke 17:1.

3. The word "offense" means: (G4625 – *skandalon*)

    - A snare or a _____

    - An injury, insult, or mistreatment that becomes a _____ in our life and hinders our relationship with others and with God.

4. Can we simply avoid offense?

Read Matthew 13:54-58.

5. Who did the people take offense with?

6. Their offense led to _____.

7. Their _____ prevented Jesus from doing mighty works there.

Facts about offense

1. Offense is one of satan's oldest tricks to cause division in God's kingdom. It provides satan with a foothold into our lives; an open door to bring destruction or to prevent healing. When we allow offense and bitterness to take root in our souls, we hinder the power of God from being released in our lives.

2. Offense itself is not deadly – if it stays in the trap. But if we pick it up and consume it and feed on it in our hearts, then we have become offended. Often this happens so subtly and so gradually that we don't even realize we have taken the bait.

3. Seeds of offense sprout into roots of bitterness. With each small offense we take, we gradually erect a fence, post by post and plank by plank. Over time, that fence causes division in our relationship with others, and in our relationship with God.[4]

Symptoms of offense

It is possible that you may not realize that you are taking the enemy's bait of offense. Take time to ponder the following symptoms of offense. They may lead you to the realization that a stumbling block has hindered you from receiving healing of your body or soul.

1. Are you angry?
   One of the signs that we have offense in our heart is ongoing anger toward someone. We may be irritated or aggravated whenever we're in this person's presence.

2. Are you keeping score?
   Another sign of offense is a tendency to keep track of offenses and compare our self to others. Read Luke 15:28-30 and notice how the "good" son reacts when his prodigal brother returns and receives forgiveness from his father.

3. Are you thinking about the offense and talking about it all the time?
   A third sign that we are harboring offense is when we feel a need or a justification to "vent"; talking about the issue with other people.

[4] John Bevere, The Bait of Satan, (Lake Mary, FL: Charisma House, 2004)

Foundation Four

God clearly commands us to forgive. Knowing the truth about what forgiveness truly is and is not will empower you to choose to forgive and receive emotional freedom.

1. First of all, forgiveness is an _____ that an offense has been committed.

2. Forgiveness does not remove or delete _____ from our lives.

   - Forgiveness will not _____ your memory, but it will remove the _____ of that memory over your life.

   - Forgiveness does not declare that what the offender did is now _____.

   - Forgiveness does not conceal the seriousness of the _____ that the offenses may have caused.

3. Forgiveness brings emotional _____.

   - _____ won't remove your pain.

   - Even the offender's _____ and _____ does not heal the wound of your soul.

   - Holding onto the offense holds you in _____ to the offense and to the offender.

   - Forgiveness is releasing a _____; releasing what you are owed. **(Matthew 6:12)**

   - When you release the debt, you are releasing your tie to the debtor, and the result is _____.

4. Forgiveness is your _____, and is not dependent upon the offender.

FORGIVE, AS YOU HAVE BEEN FORGIVEN 113

5. Jesus is our just _____ and our _____. **(Romans 12:19)**

   - Sometimes our reluctance to forgive comes when we feel that forgiveness somehow lets our offender be _____ from what they have done.
   - We do not have the right to be the _____ of justice.

   - We relinquish that right by committing that person out of our hands and into the hands of _____.

6. Forgiveness does not require a _____ of a relationship.

   - Forgiveness is always necessary, but _____ is not.

   - Reconciliation focuses on the relationship and requires both parties to be in _____ to be reconciled.

7. _____ may remain and may be necessary to prevent further wounding.

8. Forgiveness does not restore _____. Trust must be _____.

Foundation Five

God has given man free will. It is up to us to make the choice to forgive, as we have been forgiven. How do we do that?

1. First, search your heart, and ask God to reveal any offense or unforgiveness that you are holding onto.

Read Psalms 139:23-24.

   - What is the meaning of the word "wicked" (H6090 – *otseb*)?

2. Next, confess to God.

Read 1 John 1:9.

   - To confess means to openly _____ your offense or unforgiveness to God

114 GOD SAYS YES, WE SAY AMEN

- To confess means to come into _____ with God; to see unforgiveness as God sees it.

3. Now, choose to forgive.

    - Make a conscious _____ to forgive, even if the feelings of forgiveness are not yet in your heart.

    - Let go of the _____ owed to you by your offender.

    - Release your offender into the hands of _____ so that he or she will no longer have _____ over you.

    - Hand Father God your _____.

4. Receive emotional freedom!!! You have been released from the torturers!

Read John 8:36.

- When you make the choice to forgive, you are enforcing an eviction notice. The _____ has been evicted from your soul.

- You are calling on God to uproot and boot out _____ as an unwanted squatter.

- You are declaring that the real estate of your heart has a new landlord, _____, and He's been given full authority over it.[5]

---

[5]Rodney Hogue, Forgiveness, (Hayward, CA: Community of Grace, 2008)

KEEPING GOD'S WORD
Receiving It, Loving It, Living It

You have made the choice to forgive, to let go of the debt that was owed to you, and to release your offender into the hands of Jesus, the Just Judge and Defender. You have received emotional freedom.

But what about those lingering feelings of hurt or anger or guilt that were attached to the offense or unforgiveness?

1. Remember that forgiveness is an act of the will, not an emotion. Emotions come later.

    - Speak of your forgiveness out loud. There is power in what God's children declare. Your emotions are now in position to receive healing and restoration!

2. Build a godly stronghold to replace the ungodly one that was just torn down. Replace the bitterness that was uprooted with new roots of truth.

    - Meditate on God's forgiveness for you. **(Psalm 103:12)**

    - See your own debt – the debt that nailed Jesus to the cross where He endured an agonizing death. **(Romans 5:8)**

    - Meditate on the greatness of His love poured out for you, with joy! **(Hebrews 12:2)**

IN PURSUIT OF MORE

Forgive Yourself

This session of *God Says Yes, We Say Amen* deals with forgiveness – letting go of offense, canceling out all debt owed to you, and releasing the offender into the hands of Jesus. But what if the person you need to forgive is yourself? One of the enemy's most destructive lies is the one that whispers in your ear, "You are guilty as charged. You deserve to be punished. You legally owe restitution. And you certainly are not worthy of forgiveness".

That, my friend, is a lie!

How did Jesus treat the unworthy sinner while He walked on this earth? Let's look at the Word of truth …

> *Now early in the morning He came again into the temple, and all the people came to Him; and He sat down and taught them. Then the scribes and Pharisees brought to Him a woman caught in adultery. And when they had set her in the midst, they said to Him, "Teacher, this woman was caught in adultery, in the very act. Now Moses, in the law, commanded us that such should be stoned. But what do You say?" This they said, testing Him, that they might have something of which to accuse Him. But Jesus stooped down and wrote on the ground with His finger, as though He did not hear.*
>
> *So when they continued asking Him, He raised Himself up and said to them, "He who is without sin among you, let him throw a stone at her first." And again He stooped down and wrote on the ground. Then those who heard it, being convicted by their conscience, went out one by one, beginning with the oldest even to the last. And Jesus was left alone, and the woman standing in the midst. When Jesus had raised Himself up and saw no one but the woman, He said to her, "Woman, where are those accusers of yours? Has no one condemned you?"*
>
> *She said, "No one, Lord."*
>
> *And Jesus said to her, "<u>Neither do I condemn you</u>; go and sin no more."* (John 8:2-11)

Notice that the scribes and Pharisees were basing their condemnation and the required death sentence upon the law. Jesus called these men "accusers". This word, *kategoros* in the Greek, is the name given to the devil by the rabbis. And it is one of the names the Bible uses for satan, the accuser of the brethren. An accuser can be likened to a prosecuting attorney, who works for the government to uphold the letter of the law. He never exposes the defendant's good points; rather he portrays evidence of failure and strives to carry out prosecution for those failures. You can see the enemy's destructive tactics clearly exposed in this account.

But we also see the work of Jesus clearly displayed! Jesus gave the free gift of no condemnation to the adulterous. Yes, she was guilty. Yes, she broke the law, and the letter of the law stated that she deserved to be stoned to death. But Jesus, her defense attorney, represented her. The result ... she was acquitted – set free of the charge!

Let's look at another example of how Jesus treated the unworthy sinner while He walked on this earth ...

> *As Jesus went on from there, he saw a man named Matthew sitting at the tax collector's booth. "Follow me," he told him, and Matthew got up and followed him.*
>
> *While Jesus was having dinner at Matthew's house, many tax collectors and "sinners" came and ate with him and his disciples. When the Pharisees saw this, they asked his disciples, "Why does your teacher eat with tax collectors and 'sinners'?"*
>
> *On hearing this, Jesus said, "It is not the healthy who need a doctor, but the sick. But go and learn what this means: 'I desire mercy, not sacrifice.' <u>For I have not come to call the righteous, but sinners.</u>"* (Matthew 9:9-13 NIV)

Matthew was a tax collector. In his day, tax collectors were despised. They were Jews who were collecting taxes for the Romans. They were called "tax farmers", because they were allowed to collect more money than the Roman government required, and keep the rest for themselves. They were hated because the Israeli people felt they had sold out to the Romans and were not true to their Jewish heritage. They were literally excluded from the people of God.

But Jesus didn't exclude Matthew. He <u>chose him</u> to be His disciple, to be a part of His ministry, to be included within His inner circle! Jesus told the Pharisees that God desires mercy, not sacrifice. The sacrificial system was an integral part of the Old Testament system of law. The emphasis of the law was on the power of sin and exclusion. Since the Pharisees were under that system, they saw Matthew as a sinner who deserved to be excluded. But Jesus told the Pharisees that God desires mercy instead! Mercy means we do NOT get what we deserve, and is a part of the New Testament system of grace! The emphasis shifted from the power of sin and exclusion, to the power of God's love and acceptance! Jesus came to call the sinners through His mercy, through the power of His love and acceptance!

How did Jesus accomplish the exchange from condemnation to reconciliation?

Under the Old Covenant, the blood of animals poured out in sacrifice atoned for our sins. The word atone means to cover. Sin was not removed; it was just covered up. God is holy and perfect, and cannot be in communion with sinful man. Therefore, men were separated from God because of their sin.

But when Jesus established the New Covenant, everything changed. Jesus was the final Sacrificial Lamb. He was the perfect, unblemished Lamb of God, who took away the sins of the world. It is still true that sinful man cannot commune with our ultimate loving God. But Jesus fixed the problem. His blood did not just atone for our sin. His blood completely destroyed sin, effectively paying the price that we owed, so that we could be free from sin forever. As a result, we are forever separated from sin, and reconciled unto God.

Under the Old Testament, we were under condemnation. But not under the New Covenant. If we choose to accept the sacrifice by believing in Jesus and surrendering our heart to Him as our Savior, we receive acquittal … we are legally set free of the charges of all of our sins. Because of the sacrifice of Jesus, we ARE WORTHY to be in His presence. In fact, He desperately yearns for us to commune with Him!

Romans 8:1-2 (AMP) says: *There is therefore now no condemnation to those who are in Christ Jesus, who do not walk according to the flesh, but according to the Spirit. For the law of the Spirit of life in Christ Jesus has made me free from the law of sin and death.*

The power of God's love (grace) has freed us from the power of sin (law). Now that's great news!

Do you know the love of the Father through your own personal experience?

The most vital foundation for receiving the gift of worthiness from God, is to know that He loves you, that He is absolutely crazy in love with you! You are His accepted, chosen, adopted son or daughter.

> *For [the Spirit which] you have now received is not a spirit of slavery to put you once more in bondage to fear, but you have received the Spirit of adoption [the Spirit producing sonship] in [the bliss of] which we cry, Abba, Father! The Spirit Himself thus testifies together with our own spirit, assuring us that we are children of God.*
> (Romans 8:15-16 AMP)

We are the adopted children of God! In bliss, in awe, in utter joy and amazing love, we cry out "Abba, Father"! Abba is the name of endearment that Jesus used when communing with His

Father. The closest words we have in our language to equate to Abba are "Daddy" or "Papa".

Our son and his wife have their own young son. Upon his birth, Chad (our son) began to call himself "Papa" to Colton (his son). We had never used this term in our family, so it was strange at first to hear him address himself as Colton's "Papa". But as Colton grew and began to speak, one of his very first words, spoken with pure innocence and complete trust and love, was "Pa-pa". Today, when I pour out my heart to my heavenly Father, I often address Him as Papa, or Daddy, casting my cares completely upon Him, and pouring out my utter trust in Him to take care of me, much like Colton trusts his Papa to love and care for him!

But many of God's children have difficulty with this level of trust and intimacy with Father God. The problem often lies in the negative experiences through which they've lived with their earthly father. Our relationship with our own father and mother can drastically affect the way we relate to God, Who is Perfect Love! Maybe you were abandoned by your father. Maybe he was absent when you needed him. Maybe he lied to you and broke his promises. Maybe he never connected to you. Maybe you never measured up to your father's expectations. Maybe you couldn't please your father. Maybe you were fearful of him. Maybe he spoke to you or about you with damaging, hurtful words. Maybe he didn't provide for you, or protect you. Maybe he didn't love you.

Stop. Renounce the lie that Father God is like your earthly father. Go to His Word, and discover His love for you! Meditate; speak of His love for you! Receive the truth to replace the lies you have believed! Receive His love!

When someone loves you, they don't just _say_ they love you. They don't just _feel_ love for you. They also _demonstrate_ their love! *You see, at just the right time, when we were still powerless, Christ died for the ungodly. Very rarely will anyone die for a righteous man, though for a good man someone might possibly dare to die. But _God demonstrates his own love for us in this_: While we were still sinners, Christ died for us.* (Romans 5:6-8 NIV)

The enemy wants you to believe that your sinful actions will prevent God from loving you, or that you have to earn His love. More lies! Here's the truth! *Do you think anyone is going to be able to drive a wedge between us and Christ's love for us? There is no way! Not trouble, not hard times, not hatred, not hunger, not homelessness, not bullying threats, not backstabbing, not even the worst sins listed in Scripture … None of this fazes us because _Jesus loves us_. I'm absolutely convinced that nothing— nothing living or dead, angelic or demonic, today or tomorrow, high or low, thinkable or unthinkable— absolutely _nothing can get between us and God's love_ because of the way that Jesus our Master has embraced us.* (Romans 8:35-39 The Message)

So here is my final question. **Did Jesus die for you in vain? That's your choice to make!**

In Galatians 2:20-21, the Bible literally says that we have the potential to cancel out the benefit of Christ's death with our wrong-believing!

> *I have been crucified with Christ; it is no longer I who live, but Christ lives in me; and the life which I now live in the flesh I live by faith in the Son of God, who loved me and gave Himself for me. I do not set aside the grace of God; for if righteousness comes through the law, <u>then Christ died in vain.</u>"*

Have you set aside the grace of God and exchanged the truth for a lie? The truth is that Jesus took all of the punishment that we deserved to destroy sin for those who accept His sacrifice. If you are living in a state of sin-consciousness, buying the lie that you are not worthy of God's grace, then Christ died in vain.

It is truth that Jesus took the stripes on His holy back for your healing. He completed the work necessary to purchase our healing. But if we don't believe it, we will not receive it. And it is truth that Jesus shed His blood, His very life, to destroy the sin that separated you from God, so that you could be reconciled to Him. It is truth that there is now no condemnation for those who are in Christ Jesus! But if we don't believe this truth, we will not receive it.

I'd like to close this chapter with one final thought. Harboring condemnation and unworthiness (unforgiveness of self) keeps us focused on ourselves instead of on God. When we buy this destructive lie, we are actually exerting a subtle form of pride, which masquerades as humility, although it is FALSE humility. It's much more difficult to humbly receive forgiveness we don't deserve (the grace of God) than to hold onto unworthiness, cloaked in shame.

When we believe and receive forgiveness, the One who gave it is honored. God is NOT honored when we deny what Jesus did for us. He is NOT honored when we hold onto unworthiness and condemnation.

So make a choice to believe the truth, not the lie! Let go of the lie of unworthiness! And embrace your forgiven-ness!

JESUS,
HEALER OF THE WOUNDED SOUL

Beloved, I pray that you may prosper in all things and be in health, just as your soul prospers.

3 John 1:2

SESSION 9

SESSION PURPOSE

As born again children of God, our spirits are united with the Spirit of God in an eternal state of righteousness. However, our souls and bodies are not perfected. In Session 7 of *God Says Yes, We Say Amen*, we learned God's will for His children to grow in holiness through yieldedness to His Word and the Holy Spirit's unction within. In Session 8 we came to understand the completeness of God's forgiveness for us, and His command for us to forgive as He has forgiven. Both of these spiritual truths lead us to today's manna …

Sin, including unforgiveness, causes our soul to be wounded, and allows the enemy access into our souls and/or our bodies to accomplish his mission … stealing, killing, and destroying. Jesus defeated the enemy, but he didn't destroy him. We have been given authority to partner with Jesus in His mission to destroy the works of the enemy. Today you will learn just how to do that!

Foundation One

Today we will focus on wounds of the soul, and how to receive healing for those deep and festering wounds. But first we need to understand the three parts of our being.

Your <u>spirit</u> is the core of your being. It cannot be seen or felt, but it is the real you! Your spirit is eternal and will live forever. The moment you accepted Jesus' sacrifice and received Him as your Savior, your spirit was joined with the Holy Spirit, and you became reconciled to God and separated from sin. At that very moment, your born-again spirit was made as perfect and complete as it'll ever be throughout all eternity!

Read 1 Corinthians 6:17.

Your <u>soul</u> includes your mind, your intellect, your will, your emotions, your conscience, your personality, your passions, your dreams, your desires. Your soul can't be seen, but it can be felt. You can tell via your soul if you're happy or depressed, mentally worn out or sharp and ready to go, angry or frustrated or fearful or intimidated. Our souls are sanctified as we grow in relationship with Abba our loving Father, Jesus our compassionate Friend, and Holy Spirit, our nurturing Helper. In this sanctification process, we grow in submission and obedience to God. Are you choosing to yield to God or to sin, the enemy of the soul?

Your <u>body</u>, of course, is obvious. It is the house for your spirit and your soul. It can be seen and felt. Do you follow your sensual desires that may lead to sin, or do you follow the Spirit within you?

Foundation Two

When you received Jesus' salvation, your spirit was made perfect, but your soul and your body were not. When you received salvation, you were completely and eternally freed from sin. Sin **does not** affect your rightstanding with God. It **does not** affect His love for you. But sin **does** have consequences upon your soul. And the health of your soul affects the health of your body.

Read 3 John 1:2.

1. What do the words "even as" mean? (G2531 – *kathos*)

2. The health of your soul directly affects:

    - The degree of your _____

    - The _____ of your body

Foundation Three

Today we will explore two root causes of wounds of the soul.

<u>The first possible root cause of a soul wound is sin.</u> William Paul Young wrote, "Sin is its own punishment, devouring you from the inside."[6] Why? Because sin has the potential to deeply wound our soul. Sin can give demonic powers access into our soul, and sin can cause us to unknowingly forfeit our God-ordained dominion over the enemy.

Read Psalm 41:4.

1. Sin wounds the _____.

---

[6] William Paul Young, The Shack, (Los Angeles, CA: Windblown Media, 2007), 120.

Read Ephesians 4:26-27.

2. Sin gives the _____ access into your life.

   - Your sin towards _____ (i.e. anger, rage, harmful words, sexual sin)

   - Your sin towards _____ (i.e. unworthiness, guilt, condemnation, pride)

   - Other's sin towards _____ (i.e. emotional or physical abuse, neglect, abandonment, harmful words, destructive relationships)

Read Galatians 5:19-21.
The Kingdom of God referred to in Galatians 5:21 is NOT referring to going to heaven. Rather, it refers to the royal power and authority of King Jesus to rule over the kingdom of darkness. This same power and authority has been conferred upon believers. We also have dominion over all the power of the enemy, including sin!

3. When we yield to sin, we forfeit our _____ over the enemy.

A second possible root cause of a soul wound is a traumatic event or season in your life. Perhaps you have lived through a season of severe mental or emotional stress. Perhaps you have experienced an emotional upheaval in your life (i.e. death of a loved one, divorce, loss of job). Perhaps you've had a traumatic physical injury resulting from an accident, or a physical or sexual attack. In each of these instances, your soul has the opportunity to become wounded.

In the natural realm, an open wound is an access point for infection. In the spiritual realm, a soul wound is an access point for the enemy to gain a foothold into your soul and/or your body.

Foundation Four

Once a wound has taken root in the soul, it may grow into a poisonous fruit …

Emotional or Mental Dysfunction
Depression, anxiety, panic attacks, phobias, compulsive behaviors, bi-polar disorder, etc.

Physical Disease

Medical research shows that the most common root cause of physical disease is psychosomatic issues. This refers to a physical disorder that is caused or greatly influenced by emotional or mental factors. There is a direct connection between tribulations of the soul (i.e. emotional pain, fear, worry, anxiety, stress, strife) and sickness in the body.

Prevention of Healing

Have you been seeking the Healer, but haven't yet experienced the total manifestation of healing in your body? Perhaps you've been dealing with the "bad fruit" of the disease, but not the root cause. If the enemy has gained access to your soul, you need to destroy the root, which will also destroy the "bad fruit" of the disease!

Foundation Five

Jesus is our Healer. Luke 19:10 says, *"for the Son of Man has come to seek and to save that which was lost."* The word "save" in this scripture is the Greek word *sozo*, which means to heal, to make well, to restore to health, to save, to keep safe and sound, to rescue from danger, to deliver from evil. His plan for healing is inclusive … all-encompassing … perfect. His plan for healing includes healing of the spirit, the body, and the soul!

Read Psalm 147:3.

1. What does the word "brokenhearted" mean?

    - Broken (H7665 – *shabar*)

    - In heart (H3820 – *leb*)

2. What does the word "wounds" mean? (H6094 – *atstsebeth*)

Read Isaiah 61:1, 3. This is a prophetic word pointing towards the Messiah.

3. What does the word "poor" mean? (H6035 – *anav*)

4. What does the word "liberty" mean? (H1865 – *derowr*)

God doesn't just promise healing of the soul and release from bondage. He also replaces the painful effects of the woundedness with the glorious effects of healing!

5. He replaces ashes with _____!

6. He replaces mourning with the oil of _____!

7. He replaces the spirit of heaviness with the garment of _____!

Read Luke 4:16-21. The prophetic word from Isaiah 61 is fulfilled at the very onset of Jesus' ministry.

8. What does the word "oppressed" mean? (G2352 – *thrauo*)

Read Acts 10:38.

9. Jesus was anointed with _____.

10. For what purpose?

Read 1 John 3:8.

11. For what purpose was the Son of God made known to man?

Foundation Six

The Bible clearly proves that Jesus came to heal the soul as well as to heal the body. Follow the following guidelines to receive healing of your wounded soul and emotional freedom!

Step One: Acknowledge, Repent, Forgive

Ask the Holy Spirit to reveal wounds of your soul.

Acknowledge the sin or trauma that has wounded your soul.

Repent for any resentment you have held onto. Many of us have allowed bitterness, hard-heartedness, fear, self-condemnation or hatred to take up residence in our soul. Make the choice to repent, to change your mind and your heart in the area of the wound.

Forgive your offender. Let go of the debt owed to you. Release him/her into the hands of Jesus, so that he or she will no longer have power over you.

⊰⊱

Step Two: Apply the blood of the cross that has remitted all of your sin, washes away the effects of sin from your soul, and brings emotional freedom.

Read Matthew 26:28.

1. What does the word "remission" mean? (G859 – *aphesis*)

Read Ephesians 1:7.

2. What does the word "redemption" mean? (G629 – *apolytrosis*)

3. The Greek for word for "forgiveness" is *aphesis*, which is the exact same word translated as _____ in Matthew 26:28.

⊰⊱

Step Three: You have regained your dominion over the enemy. Now use your God-given authority and power to cast off the works of darkness!

Read Luke 9:1 and Luke 10:19.

4. What does the word "authority" mean? (G1849 – *exousia*)

5. What is the symbol of authority in law enforcement?

6. What does the word "power" mean? (G1411 – *dynamis*)

7. What is the symbol of power in law enforcement?

Read Romans 13:12.
Take authority over the demonic influence in your life. Cast off the power of darkness and remove the foothold of the enemy!

Say,

"I cast off the spirit of …" (i.e. rejection, abandonment, unworthiness, guilt, shame, anger, depression, anxiety, lust, control, fear, timidity)

"I break all ties with the spirit of _____ that has dominated my life."

"I cancel every agreement I have made with the spirit of _____."

"I command the spirit of _____ to remove your foothold from my life and leave me NOW, in the name of Jesus and by the power of His blood!"

✥

Step Four: Hand the soul wound and its pain to Father God. Allow Him to take it from you. Then ask Father God to replace your woundedness with His healing. If you were believing a lie, ask Him to show you the truth. Like a gift, He will replace the ashes with beauty, the sorrow with joy, the spirit of heaviness for a garment of praise!

8. Say, "Father God, I hand you …

9. Say, "What do you give me in exchange?"

✥

Repeat Steps One through Four if God reveals multiple wounds of your soul.

KEEPING GOD'S WORD
Receiving It, Loving It, Living It

1. Take time this week to reflect on the health of your soul. Ask the Holy Spirit to search your heart to reveal any wounds that reside there. Write down areas of woundedness inflicted by:

   Your sin toward others (i.e. anger, rage, harmful words, sexual sin)

   Your sin towards yourself (i.e. unworthiness, guilt, condemnation, pride)

   Other's sin towards you (i.e. emotional or physical abuse, neglect, abandonment, harmful words, destructive relationships)

   Traumatic event(s) or season(s) of your life (i.e. death of a loved one, divorce, loss of job, physical injury or accident)

2. Follow these guidelines to receive healing of your wounded soul and emotional freedom!

   Step One: Acknowledge, repent, and forgive as needed.

   Step Two: Apply the blood of the cross that has remitted all of your sin, washes away the effects of sin from your soul, and brings emotional freedom.

   Step Three: You have regained your dominion over the enemy. Now use your God-given authority and power to cast off the works of darkness!

Step Four: Hand the soul wound and its pain to Father God. Allow Him to take it from you. Then ask Father God to replace your woundedness with His healing. If you were believing a lie, ask Him to show you the truth.

Repeat Steps One through Four if God reveals multiple wounds of your soul.

IN PURSUIT OF MORE

In this session of *God Says Yes ... We Say Amen*, we have looked into the Word of truth regarding healing for the broken-hearted; healing of the soul. In Foundation Six, I shared guidelines to help you acknowledge the hurt, forgive the offender if needed, and receive healing. In the following story, I share an example of what that may look like ...

Testimony of Healing of a Soul Wound

This testimony is based upon a true story. However, I've given the woman a fictitious name to protect her privacy. Jennifer is a woman in her mid-fifties, who has never been married. She is very successful in her career, a woman of strong faith who ministers to others in need and knows God very personally and intimately. She is a woman with a strong character and personality, an excellent communicator, living a life of abundance. But during a ministry of healing directed toward the soul, Father God revealed a very deep inner wound. The wound occurred when her father died about 50 years ago. Jennifer was a very young girl at the time, only 3 years old. She barely remembered her dad, and certainly had no residual mourning or grief in her heart. She didn't even realize that her soul had been deeply wounded through her father's death.

Father God revealed the wound in her soul that was inflicted when her father abandoned her at 3 years old. When he died, he left her without a father to love her, to protect her, to provide for her, to be there for her. God revealed to her that the reason she had never married was because of this wound in her soul that caused her to believe the lie that if she allowed a man to love her, if she gave her heart in love to a man, he might abandon her too. She had closed herself off to love, because of the wound in her soul, and the lie of the enemy.

But God healed that long-standing wound. Jennifer made a choice to forgive her father for dying and abandoning her. She released him from the debt that he could never repay, the debt he owed her to be her dad, to protect her, to love her, to care for her. She handed Father God the wound of her soul, the pain of abandonment. And then she asked Him this question, "Father God, what do you have for me in exchange?"

What happened next was one of the most beautiful restorations I've ever witnessed in my years of ministry. Jennifer narrated what she was experiencing in the spiritual realm. This is what she shared.

She saw Father God come and take a little girl heart out of her chest. It was a child-sized heart. It appeared to be made of pottery, but it was completely covered with cracks. Father God removed that heart, and then He brought her a new heart. Her new heart was an adult-sized heart. It was glistening, radiant, brand-new. He took that heart and placed it in her chest, into the cavity where her old shattered heart had been. After replacing her heart, He closed her chest, and massaged it with His hands. When He lifted His hands, her chest was completely whole, without even a scar.

Jennifer had received a heart transplant! Her soul wound had been healed by the Master!

Prospering In Your Soul

In the natural realm, when we are sick, we often go to the doctor for help. Sometimes our doctor prescribes medicine to fight off an infection. But preventative care is also critically important in order to maintain a healthy life. Staying healthy requires a healthy diet, exercise, and rest.

In the spiritual realm, Jesus heals the broken-hearted. He came to set the captives free. And yes, He paid the price with His blood to heal pain and disease of the body as well as the soul. But staying healthy in our soul requires action on our part in the spiritual realm.

3 John 1:2 says, *"Beloved, I pray that you may prosper in all things and be in health, even as your soul prospers."*

The health of your body is directly related to the health of your soul. Prospering in all things (having all your needs met) is directly related to the prospering of your soul! So how do you keep your soul healthy? What are the "healthy living requirements" for your soul?

First, let me give you a visual to help you understand the magnitude of the importance of a prosperous soul. Imagine a pivot point, the very point on which something pivots or turns. Your soul is the pivot point between your spirit and your body. If your soul agrees with your spirit, you experience the life of God … you prosper in all things and are in health. Your soul gets the swing vote, the pivot point turns toward the spirit, and you receive the abundant life Jesus came to give you!

But if your soul agrees with your body, the supernatural flow of abundant life from your spirit to the physical realm stops. If your soul agrees with the issues of the flesh, that's what you will receive … sickness, pain, lack, brokenness, destruction. Your soul gets the swing vote, the pivot point turns toward the flesh, and you receive the destruction that the enemy wants you to accept!

Let's explore how your soul – your mind, your will, and your emotions -- can agree with your spirit-man; the part of you that is complete and perfect in every way.

Prospering In Your Mind

Your mind, your thoughts, and your attitudes will determine whether you experience victory and the abundant life that Jesus came to provide, or the defeat and destruction that the enemy of the world wants you to buy into. In Romans 12:2 the Apostle Paul tells us not to be conformed to this world, but to be transformed by the renewing of our mind.

The key to prospering in your mind is to continuously renew your mind with the Word of God. The Word of God has the power to transform you, to change you from one form into another (carnal-minded to spiritual-minded). It has the power to renew you, to demolish lies and wrong thinking, and to renovate your thinking in order to agree with God -- knowing His good and perfect will for you, knowing His goodness and His faithfulness! In Session 4 we learned how to meditate on the Word of God. Have you been actively contemplating, reflecting on, and pondering Scripture?

God tells us NOT to worry or be anxious! (Philippians 4:6, Matthew 6:25-34). Instead, He directs us to pray, give Him thanks, and receive His peace. In addition, He directs us to take captive any thoughts that are in opposition to His truth. As we take negative thoughts captive, we are engaging in spiritual warfare. As we take worried thoughts captive, we are spiritually overthrowing and destroying strongholds (worries are the lies of the enemy)! (2 Corinthians 10:3-5) You have a choice to worry or not to worry. Your decision is the swing vote between spirit and body!

When worries or negative thoughts attack, speak God's truth instead! There is power in the spoken Word of God! Magnify your great big God. Don't magnify the problem by constantly talking about it.

Guard what you take into your mind. Your first and most important "resource" should be the Bible! Whatever you focus on the most will predominate in your life. Be cautious of the extent of research that you do regarding the problem. Keep your focus on the solution! Keep your heart stayed on the goodness of God and His perfect will for you!

Resist confusion. Are your reading and your viewing consistent with God's Word? Is the teaching of your pastor or priest consistent with God's Word? Is all of the teaching you are listening to consistent with God's Word?

You have the swing vote. Agree with your perfected spirit! Agree with God!

Prospering In Your Will

God has given man free will, which is included within our soul. In Deuteronomy 30:19, God lays this truth out very clearly. He tells us that He sets life and death, blessings and curses before us. But He directs us to "choose life". The result of this "pro-life" choice is that both you and your descendants will live, you will love the Lord your God, you will obey His voice, and you will cling to Him! (vs. 20)

It is your choice to read God's Word, to believe it and to receive the engrafted Word into your heart. It is your choice to be teachable. It is your choice to be a doer of the Word, and not a hearer only. (James 1:21-22)

It is your choice to pray, to feed your soul with daily intimacy with God. (Hebrews 4:16) It is your choice to offer God the sacrifice of your praise, which is the fruit of your lips that thankfully acknowledge and confess and glorify His name. (Hebrews 13:15)

It is your choice to surround yourself with "believing believers" in church, in healing school, and in Bible study groups. (Hebrews 10:25) It is your choice to seek the strength of compassion that agrees with God and His will to heal, not sympathy that offers agreement with the problem (and the devil).

It is your choice to speak words of life, words of truth, words of praise. (Proverbs 18:21)

God says, "… *I set before you life and death, blessing and cursing; therefore, choose life …*" (Deuteronomy 30:19)

Prospering In Your Emotions

Our emotions are the third part of our soul. Session 10 will deal with the deadly emotion of fear, an extremely destructive force of the enemy. But today I would like to deal with two opposing emotions … discouragement and joy!

Proverbs 13:12 says, "*Hope deferred makes the heart sick, but when the desire comes, it is a tree of life.*"

Hope deferred refers to unrealized hope, hope that you haven't yet seen come to life. It's not unusual to be in a waiting period … a time of believing God for His finished work that you haven't seen manifested yet. The problem is when you allow the enemy's deception of discouragement to take you off course. Discouragement weakens your spiritual immune system, and opens the door for the enemy to wreak havoc with your faith. Questions are normal. Questions are important as we grow in our knowledge and trust in the Lord. But danger lurks when those questions lead you away from God and His truth, and into human reasoning that doesn't agree with God. If discouragement leads you into buying the demonic lie that God is not good, your heart (your soul) has become very, very sick.

You may find yourself embracing sickness, pain, or mental anguish as a gift from God. That is a devastating lie from hell. Sickness, pain, and mental anguish are gifts of the devil! It is blasphemous to attribute to God the works of the devil! God is good, all the time! The devil is bad, all the time! (John 10:10)

You may find yourself blaming yourself for not receiving healing for some reason. That's another destructive lie from the pit of hell. Your works have nothing to do with receiving healing. Jesus did all the work that was ever needed when He shed His blood for our redemption ... once and for all! When you focus on your own works, thinking that you need to do something to move God to heal you, your faith is actually hindered. But when you keep your focus on Jesus and His finished work, your faith rises up to receive God's promises.

You may even become offended with God – with your unanswered questions blocking your ability to trust in the unseen. Questions are allowed, but a lack of answers must not interrupt your communion with God. Be teachable. Continue to receive life from the engrafted Word of God.

How do you avoid the enemy's deception of discouragement and its destructive influence to your soul?

- First, be absolutely gut level honest with God. Talk to Him about your unanswered questions. Talk to Him about the struggle you're having fighting discouragement. Renounce the spirit of discouragement.

- Wait for God to respond to you. Listen. Write down His response. You may want to read from the book of Psalms until you hear your own voice and see your own heart cry. Then meditate on that Word, where there is healing for your soul.

- Give up your right to understand, and receive God's peace. (John 14:27; Philippians 4:6-7) You can only hold onto one thing at a time – the promise of God or the discouragement. You will have to drop one to embrace the other.

- Celebrate the goodness of God, which is the very bedrock of your faith. Celebrate His goodness in the very area in which you have been discouraged. If you are waiting on physical healing, praise Him for His healing, praise Him for the finished work of the cross, praise the great name Jehovah Rapha!

- Feed your soul with what God IS doing, without stumbling over what it appears that He is NOT doing. Feed your soul with testimonies of His faithfulness. Feed your soul with His benefits! (Psalm 103:1-5)

Refuse the lie of discouragement. Replace it with the Spiritual fruit of joy. Galatians 5:22-23 says, *"But the fruit of the Spirit is love, joy, peace, longsuffering, kindness, goodness, faithfulness, gentleness, self-control…"*

When we walk in the joy of the Lord, we are strengthened by the grace of God. We are empowered by the Holy Spirit to remain steadfast and immovable no matter what circumstances we may be walking through.

In about 516 BC, after the Israelites had been held captive in Babylon for 70 years, their temple was reconstructed, and the wall was finally rebuilt under the supervision of the prophet Nehemiah. Upon completion, all of the people gathered to hear the Word of God read and explained by Ezra the priest and scribe, and the Levites. After they heard the Word of God proclaimed to them, they wept in repentance. But Ezra told them to stop crying and rejoice! Here are his words, "… *Go your way, eat the fat, drink the sweet drink, and send portions to him for whom nothing is prepared; for this day is holy to our Lord. And be not grieved and depressed, for the joy of the Lord is your strength and stronghold.*" (Nehemiah 8:10 AMP)

Yes, the Israelites were deeply convicted and in a state of repentance. But that was a good thing! Father God spoke through His prophet to tell them not to be grieved or depressed, but to celebrate! The promise of their seed of joy was a harvest of strength!

Let's look at another scripture, Habakkuk 3:17-19 (AMP)
> *Though the fig tree does not blossom and there is no fruit on the vines, [though] the product of the olive fails and the fields yield no food, though the flock is cut off from the fold and there are no cattle in the stalls, Yet I will rejoice in the Lord; I will exult in the [victorious] God of my salvation!*
>
> *The Lord God is my Strength, my personal bravery, and my invincible army; He makes my feet like hinds' feet and will make me to walk [not to stand still in terror, but to walk] and make [spiritual] progress upon my high places [of trouble, suffering, or responsibility]!*

Even amidst your circumstances, rejoice in the victorious God of your salvation. He is your strength, your bravery, your army. Now that is a powerful truth! The joy of the Lord is your strength!

> Joy = Strength
> Great joy = Great strength
> Little joy = Little strength
> No joy = No strength
> You choose.

Joy is a choice, and is not conditional upon circumstances. In other words, it is not necessary to be in the midst of excellent circumstances in order to be in joy. The Apostle Paul wrote his letter to the Philippians during his two years of house arrest in Rome. This book is surnamed, "The Book of Joy". In the midst of Paul's imprisonment, he wrote about joy more than in any of his other epistles. Paul had learned through experience to choose joyousness no matter the situation. The foundation of his joy was firmly established in knowing Jesus. (Philippians 3:7-10) That joy carried him through every situation he faced with strength and steadfastness.

Rejoice in the Lord always. Again, I say rejoice. (Philippians 4:4)

Joy and faith are directly connected. When one is missing, the other will fail. As you cultivate the fruit of joy, your faith will be strengthened. As you walk in faith in the finished work of Jesus, you will experience joyous and confident expectation of His will being manifested in every situation of your life!

Romans 5:1-11, NLT
Therefore, since we have been made right in God's sight by faith, we have peace with God because of what Jesus Christ our Lord has done for us. Because of our faith, Christ has brought us into this place of undeserved privilege where we now stand, and we confidently and joyfully look forward to sharing God's glory.

We can rejoice, too, when we run into problems and trials, for we know that they help us develop endurance. And endurance develops strength of character, and character strengthens our confident hope of salvation. And this hope will not lead to disappointment. For we know how dearly God loves us, because he has given us the Holy Spirit to fill our hearts with his love.

When we were utterly helpless, Christ came at just the right time and died for us sinners. Now, most people would not be willing to die for an upright person, though someone might perhaps be willing to die for a person who is especially good. But God showed his great love for us by sending Christ to die for us while we were still sinners. And since we have been made right in God's sight by the blood of Christ, he will certainly save us *from God's condemnation. For since our friendship with God was restored by the death of his Son while we were still his enemies, we will certainly be saved through the life of his Son. <u>So now we can rejoice in our wonderful new relationship with God because our Lord Jesus Christ has made us friends of God.</u>*

Romans 15:13, AMP
May the God of your hope so fill you with all <u>joy</u> and peace in believing [through the experience of <u>your faith</u>] that by the power of the Holy Spirit you may abound and be overflowing (bubbling over) with hope.

You have the swing vote! Choose joy! Choose strength! Choose faith!

FEAR NOT, ONLY BELIEVE

But when Jesus heard it, he answered him, saying, "Do not be afraid; only believe, and she will be made well."

Luke 8:50

SESSION 10

SESSION PURPOSE

Fear is faith in the negative. Fear is another bait of satan. If we take the bait, we open ourselves to his destructive power. The purpose of this final session is to clearly contrast faith and fear, and to reveal more good news … God provides all that we need in order overcome fear and walk steadfastly in faith. We have authority as believers … *to trample on serpents and scorpions, and over all the power of the enemy, and nothing shall by any means hurt you!* (Luke 10:19)

Foundation One

The Bible commands, "Do not fear" 365 times – once for every single day of the year!!! How did Jesus help people to overcome fear?

Read Luke 8:41-42, 49-56.

1. What were Jesus' words to Jairus right after hearing of his daughter's death?

2. What actions did Jesus take to lead Jairus out of fear and into faith?

Read John 14:27.

3. What did Jesus leave to us as an inheritance?

4. What does He command us in this scripture?

Read 2 Timothy 1:7.

Fear is NOT from God. But He does give us everything we need to overcome fear!

5. He gives us the _____ of the Holy Spirit.

6. He gives us the _____ of the Father.

7. He gives us _____ from the Word of God, and Jesus is the Word made flesh. (John 1:14)

Foundation Two

Fear is faith's parallel in the negative. The chart below shows how the enemy has taken what is God's best for us – faith, and twisted it in such a way that we have faith in the negative – fear. But when the enemy's twisted truth (his lie of fear) is exposed, God's absolute truth sets us free!

FAITH	FEAR
Faith is God's creative power.	Fear is satan's destructive power.
Jesus is the author and developer of faith.	Satan is the author and developer of fear.
Faith comes by hearing the Word of God.	Fear comes by hearing the word of the enemy (the words of the world).
Faith is developed through meditating on God's truth.	Fear is developed by meditating on satan's lies (worry).

Foundation Three

We will now explore six practical strategies that will empower you to take authority over the enemy's deception of fear.

#1 - Overcome fear by trusting God!

"Trust is the fruit of a relationship in which you know you are loved."[1] You come to know God's love as you come to know Him personally. You overcome fear and step into faith as you receive the Father's love! (Review how to develop your relationship with the Father in Session 6.)

Read 1 John 4:17-18. Receive the love of the Father.

1. God's love is consummated within us through _____ and _____ with Him.

2. The perfect love of God casts out _____.

3. When fear is cast out, faith is _____.

[1] William Paul Young, The Shack, (Los Angeles, CA: Windblown Media, 2007), 126.

Read Proverbs 3:5. Remain dependent on God, not independent on your own ability.

4. Trust God. Don't try to figure out how to solve your concerns on your own. If fact, give up your right to _____!

Read 1 Peter 5:6-9. Cast your cares upon God, and leave them with Him!

5. It is _____ to give up self-control, and trust God to take care of your concerns.

6. What severe warning does this scripture give us?

7. The enemy has been _____, but not _____.

8. How do we resist the devil?

9. Fear is _____. Faith is _____!

ഔരു ഗ്രം

#2 - Overcome fear by taking fearful thoughts captive. Don't give them life through worry.

2 Corinthians 10:4-5 (AMP)
For the weapons of our warfare are not physical [weapons of flesh and blood], but they are mighty before God for the overthrow and destruction of strongholds, [Inasmuch as we] refute arguments and theories and reasonings and every proud and lofty thing that sets itself up against the [true] knowledge of God; and we lead every thought and purpose away captive into the obedience of Christ (the Messiah, the Anointed One),

1. We are fully qualified to carry out _____ that overthrows and destroys the stronghold of fear.

2. What does the word "refute" mean? (G1869 – *epairo*)

3. What are we to refute?

4. What does the word "captive" mean? (G163 – *aichmalotizo*)

5. What does the word "obedience" mean? (G5218 – *hypakoe*)

Read Philippians 4:6-8. (Review Biblical Mediation in Session 4.)

6. What are we to do INSTEAD of worrying?

7. What does God tell us to meditate on?

~~~

#3 - Overcome fear by guarding your speech.

Read Proverbs 18:21.

1. How does the fruit in your life relate to your words?

2. Ask yourself, am I magnifying _____ and His Word, or am I magnifying the _____?

> Voicing your faith cancels out fear.
> Voicing your fear cancels out faith.

Read James 1:6-8.

3. What is God's grave warning for us regarding double-mindedness?

Double-mindedness is speaking about BOTH the problem and God's truth. Words are equal to words. Thoughts are equal to thoughts. But words are FAR more powerful than thoughts. Do not buy the lie of the enemy that says that any and every worried thought that enters your mind is a sign of unbelief. Instead, take action when those worries enter your mind; take them captive and speak of God's love for you and His will for you instead. Do not entertain the worries by dwelling on them or constantly speaking of them.

> You can have faith in your heart with doubt in your mind.

#4 - Overcome fear by using the "waiting room time" in a positive way.

Don't "stare" at your circumstances – stop thinking about them, talking about them, and trying to figure them out. Instead, fix your eyes on Jesus and the work that He <u>completed</u> on the cross!

Read Hebrews 12:2-3.

1. Who is the author of your faith, and who brings it to completion?

2. If you are questioning your level of faith, or questioning if you are doing enough praying or enough reading of the Bible, or enough going to church – your focus is on the wrong person – yourself. This mindset is actually a hindrance to your faith, causing it to _____.

3. BUT, if your focus is on Jesus and all that He has completed, once and for all for you, your faith _____!

Read James 1:2-4.

4. Does God give us trials or temptations?

5. What happens within us as a result of going through trials?

6. The "waiting room time" can be a time of immense spiritual _____ and _____ healing!

7. Often the _____ person is transformed by the Holy Spirit before the manifestation of healing is seen on the _____ person.[7]

Use your time constructively, not destructively.

8. What does that look like?

9. Whatever you feed on the most will _____ in your life.

༺༻

#5 - Overcome fear by surrounding yourself with like-minded believers who will stand in faith with you.

Read Matthew 18:19-20.

1. What does it mean to agree?

2. Establish a spiritual _____, whom you can call any time that fear is attacking your faith. Don't hesitate to call your mentor to stand with you against the attack of the enemy.

3. Join a _____ with whom you can study and discuss God's Word, pray in agreement, and stand united in faith.

4. Join a _____ whose doctrinal beliefs and actions agree with God's Word.

Remember, sympathy is compassion's counterfeit, and can be deadly. (Review Session 5: "Positioned to Receive") You need strong, like-minded believers to help gird you up when you are weak.

5. Sympathy agrees with the problem, and _____ it.

6. Compassion agrees with God, and _____ the receiver.

[7]Charles Price, The Real Faith for Healing, (Gainesville, FL: Bridge Logos Publishers, 2009), 89.

#6 - Overcome fear by praising and worshipping God!

As you make the choice to enter into praise, you enter into the presence of the Lord. He inhabits the praises of His people! Praise changes the atmosphere. It is a dynamic, powerful force that defeats the enemy!

Read Romans 4:20-21.

When Abraham praised and glorified God:

1. He was _____ in faith.

2. He did not waver in _____.

3. He was fully convinced that what God had _____ He was also able to perform!

Read Psalm 34:1-4.

4. As we continually offer God our praise; as we magnify and exalt His holy name, He hears us, and delivers us from all of our _____.

KEEPING GOD'S WORD
Receiving It, Loving It, Living It

1. Do your words magnify God and His Word, or the problem you're fighting, or both? If you discover that you have been speaking the words of the world (the diagnosis, the symptoms, the treatment, the prognosis), make a decision not to cross certain lines with your tongue.

    - Who will you talk to?

    - What will you share?

    - What will you say to the rest of the people who care about you?

2. How are you using your "waiting room time"?

    - What are the spiritually constructive uses of your time?

    - What activities do you fill your time with that are not building you up?

    - What changes can you make?

3. Establish a spiritual mentor. Make sure that this person is a "believing believer", and that they are willing to mentor you. Let them know you seek compassion and strength, not sympathy.

    - Who is your mentor?

    - Do you commit to call them when you are in need?

    - Do you make the choice to be teachable?

IN PURSUIT OF MORE

Jesus – Faith; Satan – Fear

Jesus is the author and the finisher of our faith. (Hebrews 12:2) He is the Way, and the Truth, and the Life. (John 14:6) God's best for us is to live in faith in His truth. His part in our abundance of life and redemption is complete; our part is to simply believe in His finished work. (Ephesians 2:8) He is pleased when we live in faith. (Hebrews 11:6) He is not pleased when we shrink back in fear. (Hebrews 10:38) We can have faith in God and His Word because He cannot lie. (Titus 1:2) His word is true, and He is faithful.

The enemy is a deceiver and an accuser, and is the father of lies. These words were spoken by Jesus to those who were to kill him, *"You are of your father the devil, and the desires of your father you want to do. He was a murderer from the beginning, and does not stand in the truth, because there is no truth in him. When he speaks a lie, he speaks from his own resources, for he is a liar and the father of it.* (John 8:44)

The enemy is a liar, and his lies bring fear. If we believe his lies and receive the fear, our faith is weakened or maybe even destroyed.

God — Truth — Faith — Life
Satan — Lies — Fear — Death
Which will you believe and receive?

My Testimony of Overcoming Fear

When I was originally diagnosed with stage-four melanoma, I was immediately gripped by fear and lying symptoms that spawned even greater fear. Looking back, I know that the enemy was feeding me his bait and just waiting for me to take it. And I did – hook, line, and sinker – because of ignorance. The fear was dark and oppressive. It weighed heavy on my soul like the lead blanket that you are draped with before getting dental x-rays. It was constant, heavy, suffocating, life sucking, destructive, cancerous. I couldn't eat. I couldn't sleep. I could barely breathe.

I received salvation just six days after I was given the diagnosis of stage-four melanoma and gripped with satan's fear. When I prayed the prayer of salvation, I surrendered my life to God, and received His life in exchange! Then my relationship with my Father began. I didn't know Him well at first. I didn't understand His Word or His will for me. I certainly wasn't strong in faith. I just showed up, and He met me right where I was. Immediately and spontaneously, the blanket of oppressive fear lifted. Philippians 4:7 came to pass in my life. I went to my Father with my needs and simply surrendered control of my health to Him. Then His amazing peace rose up within me, assertively taking the place of the death-gripping fear!

Something happened to me in the spiritual realm. I was rescued from the demonic captivity of fear, and placed in a "safe house" with peace standing guard over my mind and heart. God was on my side! And if God is for us, who can be against us? (Romans 8:31)

I have come to recognize patterns in the enemy's attacks of fear, and will expose them to you so that you too are aware and on the defensive.

Satan attempts to lure us into fear using the bait of a medical test of some sort. As we await the test, he whispers worried thoughts into our mind and waits for us to give those worried thoughts life by speaking about them and magnifying his negative, yet ungrounded lies.

Another demonic fear bait is what I call a "lying symptom" or a "spirit of pain". You may actually feel a symptom or pain in your physical body that causes you to fear the very worst. In my case, as soon as I was given the cancer diagnosis, I was attacked with symptoms and pain … and massive fear that came right along with those lies. The pain and symptoms were very real, but not real at all. When I took authority by speaking the truth of God's Word, in the authority of the name of Jesus, they had to bow down and retreat. (James 4:7)

It seems like whenever you are fighting something in your life or your body, you come across people or hear stories about others who are in a similar battle. The problem is that their results may not be good. As a result, your faith is shaken and that lure of fear draws close, waiting for you to receive the deception.

Another bait the enemy uses is reports – bad reports or good ones! A bad report (one that doesn't agree with God's report) spurns fear and dread and terror if we give way to the accuser and his lies. But we don't have to give an inch to fear! We have God's report … saved, healed, and delivered! No matter what the medical word is, God's Word supersedes it! Whose report will you believe? (Isaiah 53:1, 4-5)

But I've also experienced huge attacks of fear after a GOOD report. The oppressor does not want God to be glorified. He wants us in a position of cowardice to him, so that we aren't in a position to bring God glory. He wants the world to question the goodness of God. Therefore, he attempts to deceive us into taking his fear bait after getting a good report so that we will take back the sickness rather than keep our healing.

That is exactly what happened to me …

It was the summer of 2002. I had just received my amazing divine healing of stage-four melanoma. I was declared cancer free, with no need for treatment. That's when the attack came. The original diagnosis of stage-four melanoma showed disease in my groin, my lower and upper abdomen, and in my neck. Exploratory surgery and lymph node excisions had confirmed that I had no cancer in my groin or abdomen, but I had no such confirmation regarding the melanoma detected by the CT and PET scans in my neck. That's where the symptoms showed up. My neck hurt. I was constantly feeling the nodules in the lymph nodes of my neck. Worry and fear attacked with a vengeance along with the haunting symptoms.

Then God gave me a rhema word that enabled me to conquer satan's relentless attack of lying symptoms. He gave me the word in my sleep. When I awoke on this particular day, "Deuteronomy 1" was in my mind, and it would not go away, kind of like a melody stuck in my head. I had never read the book of Deuteronomy. At that time, I hadn't read much of the Old Testament at all. But this word from God saved my life.

The first chapter of Deuteronomy tells of a time when the Israelites were in the desert, and grew impatient and frustrated and filled with fear in the midst of their wilderness experience. God had instructed them to take possession of the hill country of the Amorites, encouraging them not to be afraid or discouraged (vs. 21).

Twelve spies went ahead to check out the situation before actively carrying out God's direction for possessing the land of the Amorites. Ten of the twelve came back with their focus on the "bad report", speaking with fear about the Amorite people who were greater and stronger than they were, and speaking of their great and fortified cities (vs. 28).

God spoke to them through Moses, *"Do not be terrified; do not be afraid of them. The Lord your God, who is going before you, will fight for you, as he did for you in Egypt, before your very eyes, and in the desert. There you saw how the Lord your God carried you, as a father carries his son, all the way you went until you reached this place. In spite of this, you did not trust in the Lord your God, who went ahead of you on your journey, in fire by night and in a cloud by day, to search out places for you to camp and to show you the way you should go"*. (Deuteronomy 1:29-33 NIV)

Remember, twelve spies went to scope out the hill country of the Amorites. Two of those spies, Joshua and Caleb, came back with their focus on the "good report", the land of milk and honey – the amazing promised land God had told them about! Joshua and Caleb, who had kept their eyes and words and heart on God's good report, were the only people from their entire generation that actually made it to the promised land! Every single other person from their generation died in the wilderness!

As I read and reread and meditated on this chapter of Deuteronomy, the Lord revealed to me the parallel between the Israelites in the wilderness and my own life. The Lord had delivered the Israelites out of slavery, and had constantly protected them and provided for their needs. He parted the Red Sea for them, allowing it to close over their enemies. He fed them manna from heaven, and then quail when they were complaining of the manna. He gave them water from a rock. He showed them their way with a cloud by day and a fire by night. But still they grumbled and complained with doubt, fear, and unbelief.

And here I was, doing the same thing. God had given me my miracle. He had confirmed my healing. But I was still in fear, doubting God's perfect healing in my body. Remember the 10 spies who focused on the bad report, and never received their promise? I realized that if I continued in fear, I might lose my promise – my healing. But God is so very good! I recognized His loving warning, loud and clear. I took the words from Deuteronomy, and began to meditate on them. This was (is) His promise to me:

> *"Cindy, don't be terrified, don't be afraid of recurring cancer. The Lord your God, who is going before you, will continue to fight for you, just as He did when He first healed your body of cancer before your very eyes. You saw how the Lord your God carried you, the way a father carries his child. He will continue to go ahead of you on your blessed journey."* (Personal paraphrase of Deuteronomy 1:29-33)

The symptoms in my neck gradually disappeared. I had defeated fear! I had defeated satan!

※

Eight years later, the enemy attacked again. During a regular physical exam, my doctor discovered a mass in my neck. I'd like to say that I didn't waver, that fear was long-since dead and buried. But that wasn't the case. Fear was once again fueled, but I fought against the spiritual attack with spiritual warfare.

What did I do? I did exactly what we learned about in this session.

I put my trust in my great big God. I meditated on His love for me constantly. When I was attacked by fear, His manifest love would literally wash that fear off of me! It was like taking a shower and washing off filth! During that season, God gave me this amazing promise about trusting Him and knowing His love for me …

"Cindy, because you have set your love upon Me, therefore I will deliver you. I will set you on high, because you know and understand My name, you have a personal knowledge of My mercy, love, and kindness, you trust and rely on Me, knowing I will never forsake you, no, never! You shall call upon Me, and I will answer you. I will be with you in trouble. I will deliver you and honor you. With long life will I satisfy you, and show you My salvation!"
(Personal paraphrase of Psalm 91:14-16 AMP)

I did my best to take worried thoughts captive, and I replaced the enemy's voice of worry and fear with the voice of my Father and His Word of Truth. I remember speaking God's promises over my body in words like this, "Father, I have a good report … because I have YOUR report! And the doctor's report simply has to line up with it!" "Father, I thank you that by the stripes of Jesus I WAS healed, by the stripes of Jesus I AM healed, and by the stripes of Jesus I will STAY healed!"

I did not magnify the problem by talking about it. I was leading a weekly healing class, and never told the people of the fear I was facing until I came back with my testimony! I didn't even tell my family until I was scheduled for surgery, and then I was very cautious about what I shared. I clearly entreated them not to talk about any worries among themselves, or with others … and they honored my request.

I was in a "waiting room time" for six months. But God encouraged me through His Word in James 1:2-4. He showed me that in the process of the trial that I was living through, He was growing me up and maturing me, which would result in His plan and purpose for my life being released in an even greater measure! And it was! At the conclusion of my "waiting room time" I received my good report. And that very summer I drafted a new book entitled, *Healed For Life: How to Keep Your Healing*. I had learned so very much during that season, which is now ministering to people all over the world through my book!

What did I fill my time with? I continued to teach healing. I continued to minister and pray for those in need. I began research and planned for the writing of my new book on how to keep your healing.

I needed spiritual support during that season. I leaned on Jenn, my spiritual mentor. I confided in my pastor and received prayer support. My husband stood firm with me in faith. Our ministry team who supported our healing ministry agreed with me in faith for God's perfect will to be manifest in my body once again.

I constantly strengthened my faith and overcame fear through praise and worship to my Healer, my Lord, my Redeemer!

I did have surgery to remove that mass, along with my thyroid. The pathology report came back five days post-surgery. There was **no evidence of malignancy** in the mass, in my thyroid, or in the surrounding lymph nodes. Once again, God's report was verified by the doctor's report. I wasn't surprised, but I was certainly filled with joy! The very evening after receiving this good report, I taught at our weekly healing meeting. I was determined not to let the enemy stop God's Word from going forth. Five days after having a thyroidectomy, with a weak voice, but a strong anointing, God's Word was poured out … and He was glorified!

QUESTIONS AND ANSWERS

Session 1
Yes, It IS God's Will To Heal!

Foundation One

1. Griefs (H2483 – *choliy*) **sickness, disease, weakness, distresses**

2. Sorrows (H4341 – m*ak'ob*) **pain – mental, emotional, or physical**

3. Transgressions (H6588 – *pasha*) **known or unknown sin**

4. Iniquities (H5771 – *'avon*) **intentional sin, willful disobedience, perversity, depravity**

5. Chastisement (H4148 – *muwcar*) **penalty or price**

6. Peace (H7965 – *shalowm*) **safety, welfare, prosperity, health, completeness, soundness in body, nothing missing and nothing broken, tranquility, contentment**

7. Healed (H7495 – *rapha*) **cure, heal, repair, thoroughly make whole, restore to normal**

8. How many were brought to Jesus? **many**

9. How many did He heal? **all who were sick**

10. What was the ultimate purpose for His healing? **to fulfill the prophetic word**

11. Took (G2983 – *lambanō*) **to take in order to carry away; to remove**

12. Infirmities (G769 – *astheneia*) **weakness or frailty in body or soul**

13. Bore (G941 – *bastazō*) **to take up in order to bear**

14. When did we die to sin and gain access to a life of righteousness? **When we chose to accept Jesus' sacrifice through our belief in Him, and our declaration of that belief**

15. What is the meaning of the word "healed" (G2390 – *iaomai*)? **physical healing, curing of the human body**

Session 2
God's Perfect Will for You!

Foundation Two

1. The Son can do nothing of Himself, but only **what He sees the Father do.**

2. We have been delivered from **the power of darkness** and transferred into **the Kingdom of the Son of His love!**

3. Jesus is the **exact likeness** of the unseen God!

4. Jesus is the sole expression of the **glory of God**.

5. He is the perfect imprint and the very image of God's **nature**.

6. If Jesus healed all when He ministered in flesh and blood on this earth 2000 years ago, He still heals today! He is the same, **yesterday**, **today**, and **forever**!

Foundation Four

1. When do you receive salvation? **when you confess with your mouth the Lord Jesus, and believe in your heart that God has raised Him from the dead.**

2. What is the meaning of the word saved in verse 9? (G4982 – *sozo*) **saved, healed, delivered, made whole**

3. People perish from **lack** of knowledge.

4. People perish from not **receiving** knowledge.

5. People perish from not **applying** knowledge.

6. Satan is the god of this world and has **blinded** unbelievers.

7. But satan is not our god! We are **in** the world, but not **of** the world! God is our God!

8. Satan's job description: **steal, kill, destroy**

9. Jesus's job description: **that we may have and enjoy life to the full, until it overflows**

10. God sets before us life and **death**, blessings and **curses**.

11. Who gets to choose? **We do!**

Session 3
Faith ... Simply Believe!

Foundation One

What is the deeper meaning of the following words?

1. Faith – **being fully persuaded of truth**

2. Substance – **foundation**

3. Hope – **confident, joyous expectation**

4. Evidence – **proof, confirmation**

5. Things not seen – **things not revealed to the senses**

Foundation Two

1. How did Abraham act in faith? **He obeyed and left his homeland.**

2. Did he understand God's plan and how it would be accomplished? **No! He didn't know or trouble his mind about God's plan that he didn't fully understand.**

3. What did Sarah think of God's promise? **She considered God reliable, trustworthy, and true to His word.**

4. What was the result of their faith? **The promise God had given them came to pass. Abraham became the father of many nations.**

5. What did Abraham do when then the situation was utterly hopeless? **He hoped in faith anyway.**

6. Did Abraham and Sarah have reason to doubt God's promise? **Yes! Abraham was impotent and Sarah was barren, and they were long past their childbearing years.**

7. How was his faith strengthened? **By giving praise and glory to God.**

8. Why did he NOT doubt God? **He was fully satisfied and assured that God was able and mighty to keep His word and to do what He had promised.**

Foundation Three

1. The opposite of being humble is being full of **pride**.

2. The opposite of being in submission to God is being in **control** yourself.

3. The opposite of being dependent upon God is being **independent**.

4. First, **submit** to God. THEN **resist** the devil, and he will flee!

5. It is **humbling** to give up control, cast your cares on God, and simply trust Him!

6. What does it mean to "lean on your own understanding"? **To rely on your own insight, to reason out the problem or situation, to plan, research, etc.**

7. All scripture is given by **inspiration** of God.

8. The word of God is **alive** and **powerful**.

Session 4
Great Faith

Foundation One

1. What is a "mountain"? **Any insurmountable obstacle.**

2. Jesus tells us not to doubt in our **heart**.

3. What is our part in receiving the answer to our prayer? **Speak to the mountain. Believe in your heart that you receive.**

4. When does Jesus tell to believe? **When you pray.**

5. What is the promise given to us about the prayer of faith? **You will have whatever you ask when you pray in faith.**

6. According to Strong's Concordance, the word receive (G2983 - *lambano*) means **have taken**.

7. Now read Mark 11:24 with this deeper meaning unveiled … "Therefore I say to you, whatever things you ask when you pray, believe that you **have taken** them, and you will have them."

Foundation Two

1. Logos is the **written** Word of God.

2. Rhema is the **spoken or revealed** Word of God.

3. What are the 3 Greek words for the word "nothing" in this scripture? **no thing rhema**

4. In John 15, Jesus tells us that He is the **Vine** and we are the **branches**.

5. What is the variable in this promise? **If we ask according to His will, agreement with His own plan.**

6. What is the guarantee in this promise? **He listens and hears us, and we know we have granted us as our present possessions the requests made of Him.**

7. Where does our confidence come from? **Our confidence comes from knowing His will!**

Foundation Three

1. What is the purpose of rain and snow? **To water the earth, to make it bring forth and sprout**

2. Compare the Word of God to the rain and the snow. **It produces the fruit of the words we speak.**

3. The Word of God shall not return **void (canceled) without producing any effect, or useless.**

4. It shall **accomplish** that which I speak.

5. It shall **prosper** in the thing for which I sent it.

6. God creates the **fruit** of our **lips**.

7. What is the meaning of the word "peace" (H7965 – *shalowm*)? **Completeness, safety, soundness in body, health, nothing missing or broken, welfare, prosperity, tranquility, contentment**

8. What is the meaning of the word "heal" (H7495 – *rapha*)? **Cure, heal, repair, thoroughly make whole, restore to normal**

9. Whose words does verse 9 refer to? **The Word of God**

10. Where are those words located? **In our mouth**

11. What is the promise God gives us in verse 12? **He is alert and active, watching over His word to perform it.**

Foundation Four

1. Read all of these scriptures from Proverbs 4, and underline the word "live" or "life" in each scripture.

2. What is the meaning of the word "life" (H2416 – *chay*)? **A living thing, physical life**

3. Make a list of at least 5 directions found in these verses regarding God's Word in relation to life (*chay*)?
   **1. Hold fast, keep the Word
   2. Hear, receive the Word
   3. Take firm hold, do not let go, guard the Word
   4. Attend, consent, submit to the Word
   5. Keep the Word at the center of your heart**

4. What is the result of keeping His Word in the midst of your heart? **Life, healing, health**

5. What is the meaning of the word "health" (H4832 – *marpe*)? **Medicine, a cure**

Session 5
Positioned to Receive

Foundation One

1. Meditate means: **To contemplate, to reflect upon, to focus your thoughts upon, to ponder**

2. <u>Fear</u> is developed as you meditate on the problem.

3. <u>Faith</u> is established as you meditate on the Word of God.

Foundation Two

1. How do you guard your heart? **Be cautious of what you feed it. Put contrary talk far away from you!**

2. Words of life produce the fruit of <u>healing</u> and <u>health</u>.

3. Words of death produce the fruit of **sickness** and **pain**.

4. Magnify **God** and his **promises**.

5. Don't magnify the **problem**!

6. As you magnify God, you **minimize** the problem.

Foundation Three

1. As God's children, we don't **deny** the medical report.

2. But we DO deny it's **right** to **exist** in our body!

Foundation Four

1. It's absolutely fine to seek medical help and to take medicine. But put your faith in **God**.

2. **Pray** for your doctor.

3. **Pray** over your medical treatment.

Foundation Five

1. God's Word brings **peace** and God's **creative** power.

2. Research fuels **fear** and the enemy's **destructive** power.

Foundation Six

1. Who should we be looking unto? **Jesus!**

2. Jesus is the **author** and **finisher** of our faith!

3. Keep your focus on Jesus, and His finished work, not on your own works. Your faith will be **strengthened**.

4. When you focus on yourself … your works … your strength … it is a **hindrance** to your faith.

Foundation Seven

1. Sympathy is **agreement** with you in the problem.

2. Sympathy **nourishes** the problem and it is magnified.

3. Sympathy acknowledges the problem, but cannot offer **solutions**.

4. Sympathy offers **coping skills** rather than deliverance.

5. Sympathy is compassion's **counterfeit**.

6. Compassion is **practical**, **biblical**, and **bold**.

7. The focus and anchor of compassion is **Jesus**, and His will to heal!

8. What does the word "agree" mean? (G4856 – *symphoneo*) **Harmonize together**

9. You need to have others in agreement with you regarding **healing**, not the disease! You need others who will be **strong** with you, not pity you in your weakness! You need others who will speak **God's truth** over you, not talk with you about the problem!

Foundation Eight

1. Whatever you feed on the most will **predominate** in your life.

2. You **become** what you **behold**.

Foundation Nine

1. The anti-venom for confusion is **trust** in **God**.

2. God is the author of **peace**.

3. Who is the author of confusion? **The enemy**

Session 6
Seek the Healer

Foundation One

1. As you become rooted and grounded in the love of God ... **the seeds of the truth of His love take root and become firmly established in your heart.**

2. The width of God's love ... **the magnitude; the greatness of size or extent**

3. The length of His love ... **the infinitude; the boundlessness**

4. The depth of His love ... **the unfathomability; incapability to fathom or understand**

5. The height of His love ... **the summit; the highest degree; the fullest development**

6. To <u>know</u> the love of God means ... **to personally experience His love**

Foundation Two

1. What is God's plan for you? **To take care of you, not abandon you, to give you the future you hope for.**

2. What is His plan conditional upon? **You must call on Him, come and pray to Him, come looking for Him, get serious about finding Him.**

3. What does the word "abide" mean? (G3306 – *meno*) **To dwell permanently with Him, to live in Him, to be vitally united to Him.**

4. What is God's condition for "fruit-bearing" in us? **Abiding in Jesus.**

Foundation Three

1. What does the word "conformed" mean? (G4964 – *syschematizo*) **pressed into the mold of the world**

2. What does the word "transformed" mean? (G3339 – *metamorphoo*) **change from one form to another, like the metamorphosis of a caterpillar into a butterfly**

3. What does the word "renewing" mean? (G342 – *anakainosis*) **renovation; remodel; old thought patterns demolished and completely remodeled**

4. What does the word "prove" mean? (G1381 – *dokimazo*) **to test, examine, and recognized as genuine after examination**

5. What is the meaning of the word "inspiration"? (G2315 – *theopneustos*) **God-breathed**

6. Scripture is profitable for:

    Doctrine – **instruction**

    Reproof – **conviction**

    Correction – **restoration to right state; improvement of life or character**

    Instruction in righteousness – **state of being, not state of doing; we are righteous through Christ**

7. The Word **completes and equips** us!

Foundation Four

1. When and where did Jesus pray? **In the morning before sunrise; in a deserted, isolated place**

2. What happened before this prayer time? **Jesus taught in the synagogue, cast out demons, healed Peter's mother-in-law, healed all who came to him from the village after sunset**

3. What did Jesus do right after His prayer time? **Went into the next village(s) to preach**

4. Do not **worry**.

5. Pray about **every** thing and **any** thing.

6. Give **thanks**.

7. We get His **peace** that will **guard** our heart and mind.

8. Why can we come boldly and confidently before the very throne of grace in prayer? **Because of Jesus' sacrifice – we are made righteous!**

9. When we pray in our time of need, we obtain God's **mercy** and find His **grace**.

10. What is the meaning of the word "mercy"? (G1656 – *eleos*) **We don't get what we deserve for our failures – judgment, punishment**

11. What is the meaning of the word "grace"? (G5485 – *charis*) **We get what we don't deserve – unmerited favor, righteousness, wholeness, healing, peace**

Foundation Five

1. Abraham did NOT **waver** at the promise of God through unbelief.

2. Rather, he was **strengthened** in faith as he gave praise and glory to God!

3. What was Abraham fully convinced of? **That what God had promised He was also able to perform.**

4. Praise God **continually**.

5. What is the meaning of the word "magnify"? (H-1431 – *gadal*) **To make large. God is bigger than the problem!**

6. What is the meaning of the word "exalt"? (H-7311 – *ruwm*) **To make high. God is higher than the problem!**

7. What is the result when we praise God? **He hears us and delivers us from all our fears. (Fear is the opposite spiritual force from faith.)**

8. Forget not all His **benefits**!

9. A sacrifice involves giving God your **best**, no matter what the circumstances.

10. A sacrifice of praise **costs** you something! (your time, your focus, your comfort)

11. Praise is an act of your **will**. Do not allow your **emotions** to dictate your decision to praise.

12. Praising in the midst of the battle requires **faith**.

Session 7
Godly Living

Foundation One

1. Our old man was **crucified** with Jesus, so that we should no longer be **slaves** of sin.

2. For one who dies is **freed** from sin.

3. We too now live in **unbroken fellowship** with God, because of the sacrifice of our Savior!

4. Why doesn't sin have dominion (control) over us any more? **We are no longer under the law of sin and death, but under grace!**

5. Sin is deprived of its **power** over all who accept Jesus' sacrifice.

6. At that very moment, our born-again spirit was created in a state of **righteousness**.

Foundation Two

1. Righteousness is the gracious **gift** of God whereby all who **believe** in the Lord Jesus Christ are brought into right relationship with God.

2. It is unattainable by our **obedience** to any law, or our own **merit**, or our **works**.

3. Righteousness is based entirely upon receiving what **Jesus** has done.

4. It is not something we **have**. It is something we **are**.

5. Our **spirit** is perfected in this state of righteousness.

6. Our **soul** and **body** are not made perfect at the time of salvation.

7. Holiness is not a gift from God, but a decision of **obedience** in man by his own free will.

8. God supplies the **grace**, man supplies the submission and obedience to the Word of God, and **holiness** is the result

9. Holiness is something we **develop**. It is a **process**.

Foundation Three

1. What does the word "sanctify" mean? (G37 – *hagiazo*) **separated from profane things, consecrated unto God, purified, made holy**

2. Do you sanctify yourself? **No, God Himself sanctifies you.**

3. What parts of us will be preserved blameless (carefully attended and taken care of)? **Spirit, soul, and body**

4. What does Jesus pray we will be sanctified through? **The Word**

5. Unless we're shaped by the **Word**, we'll be shaped by the **world**.

6. The water of the word sanctifies and cleanses us from the **uncleanness** of life.

7. The Word of God cleanses us, woos us, draws us nearer to God. The **closer** you come to God, the less junk you can take with you!

8. We are transformed (sanctified) by beholding the glory of the Lord in the **Word of God.**

9. We **become** what we **behold**.

10. Sanctification is when we let God **make us more like Him**.

11. This happens by **coming to know Him**.

Foundation Five

1. How was the New Covenant ratified? **Through the shed blood of Jesus**

2. What was the result of the New Covenant? **The remission of sins**

3. What does the word "redemption" mean? **Our ransom was paid in full, liberated, freed, delivered**

4. The word "forgiveness" in this scripture is the exact same Greek word as the word **remission.**

Foundation Six

1. When we make mistakes and yield to the enemy instead of God, we need to run back into the arms of Abba in a position of **humility** and **surrender** to His grace.

2. Repentance is the result of a truly **surrendered** heart. It is a result of renewing your mind to God, His goodness, His forgiveness – and then **change happens**.

3. Turning from sin to God is the result of **repentance**.

4. In this process of surrendering to the grace of God and repentance, the enemy's access to your soul or your body is **revoked**!

5. We are confident in our God because we know our position of **righteousness** in Christ.

6. We grow in **holiness** as we come close to Abba with a heart of surrender and yieldedness to His loving voice of conviction and encouragement.

7. We keep His Word when we **believe in Jesus**, and **love one another**.

8. What is God's promise for us as a result? **We receive from Him whatever we ask.**

Session 8
Forgive, As You Have Been Forgiven

Foundation One

1. What does the word "redemption" mean? **Our ransom was paid in full, liberated, freed, delivered**

2. The word "forgiveness" in this scripture is the exact same Greek word as the word **remission**.

Foundation Three

1. Jesus uses this parable to teach about forgiveness. The servant owed the king 10,000 talents, which is equal to about $10,000,000! What did the king do when his heart was filled with compassion? **He released him and forgave Him, cancelling the debt.**

2. That same servant was owed about a hundred denarii by one of his peers, which is equal to about $20! What did he choose to do? **He was unwilling to give the man extra time to pay his debt. He had him put in prison until he paid his debt.**

3. The word "offense" means: (G4625 – *skandalon*)

    - A snare or a **trap**

    - An injury, insult, or mistreatment that becomes a **stumbling block** in our life and hinders our relationship with others and with God.

4. Can we simply avoid offense? **No, offenses will come.**

5. Who did the people take offense with? **Jesus!**

6. Their offense led to **unbelief**.

7. Their **unbelief** prevented Jesus from doing mighty works there.

Foundation Four

1. First of all, forgiveness is an **acknowledgment** that an offense has been committed.

2. Forgiveness does not remove or delete **offenses** from our lives.
   - Forgiveness will not **erase** your memory, but it will remove the **power** of that memory over your life.
   - Forgiveness does not declare that what the offender did is now **okay**.
   - Forgiveness does not conceal the seriousness of the **hurt** that the offenses may have caused.

3. Forgiveness brings emotional **freedom**.
   - **Revenge** won't remove your pain.
   - Even the offender's **remorse** and **repentance** does not heal the wound of your soul.
   - Holding onto the offense holds you in **bondage** to the offense and to the offender.
   - Forgiveness is releasing a **debt**; releasing what you are owed.
   - When you release the debt, you are releasing your tie to the debtor, and the result is **emotional freedom**.

4. Forgiveness is your **choice**, and is not dependent upon the offender.

5. Jesus is our just **Judge** and our **Defender**.
   - Sometimes our reluctance to forgive comes when we feel that forgiveness somehow lets our offender be **discharged** from what they have done.
   - We do not have the right to be the **enforcer** of justice.
   - We relinquish that right by committing that person out of our hands and into the hands of **Jesus**.

6. Forgiveness does not require a **restoration** of a relationship.
   - Forgiveness is always necessary, but **reconciliation** is not.
   - Reconciliation focuses on the relationship and requires both parties to be in **agreement** to be reconciled.

7. **Boundaries** may remain and may be necessary to prevent further wounding.

8. Forgiveness does not restore **trust**. Trust must be **earned**.

Foundation Five

1. First, search your heart, and ask God to reveal any offenses or unforgiveness that you are holding onto.

    - What is the meaning of the word "wicked" (H6090 – *otseb*)? **Pain, sorrow, idol**

2. Next, confess to God.

    - To confess means to openly **acknowledge** your offense or unforgiveness to God

    - To confess means to come into **agreement** with God; to see unforgiveness as God sees it.

3. Now, choose to forgive.

    - Make a conscious **choice** to forgive, even if the feelings of forgiveness are not yet in your heart.

    - Let go of the **debt** owed to you by your offender.

    - Release your offender into the hands of **Jesus** so that he or she will no longer have **power** over you.

    - Hand Father God your **hurt**.

4. Receive emotional freedom!!! You have been released from the torturers!

    - When you make the choice to forgive, you are enforcing an eviction notice. The **enemy** has been evicted from your soul.

    - You are calling on God to uproot and boot out **bitterness** as an unwanted squatter.

    - You are declaring that the real estate of your heart has a new landlord, **Jesus**, and He's been given full authority over it.

Session 9
Jesus, Healer of the Wounded Soul

Foundation Two

1. What do the words "even as" mean? (G2531 – *kathos*) **In proportion to, in the degree that**

2. The health of your soul directly affects:

   - The degree of your **prosperity**

   - The **health** of your body and soul

Foundation Three

1. Sin wounds the **soul**.

2. Sin gives the **devil** access into your life.

   - Your sin towards **others**

   - Your sin towards **yourself**

   - Other's sin towards **you**

3. When we yield to sin, we forfeit our **dominion** over the enemy.

Foundation Five

1. What does the word "brokenhearted" mean?

   - Broken (H7665 – *shabar*) **broken in pieces, shattered, crushed, wrecked, quenched**

   - In heart (H3820 – *leb*) **inner man, soul, mind, will, understanding**

2. What does the word "wounds" mean? (H6094 – *atstsebeth*) **pain, hurt, injury, sorrow**

3. What does the word "poor" mean? (H6035 – *anav*) **weak, afflicted, lowly**

4. What does the word "liberty" mean? (H1865 – *derowr*) **release from bondage or imprisonment**

5. He replaces ashes with **beauty**!

6. He replaces mourning with the oil of **joy**!

7. He replaces the spirit of heaviness with the garment of **praise**!

8. What does the word "oppressed" mean? (G2352 – *thrauo*) **broken in pieces, shattered, broken by clamaity**

9. Jesus was anointed with **the Holy Spirit and with power**.

10. For what purpose? **To do good and to heal all who were oppressed by the devil!**

11. For what purpose was the Son of God made known to man? **That He might destroy the works of the devil!**

Foundation Six

1. What does the word "remission" mean? (G859 – *aphesis*) **release from penalty, pardon of sin, letting them go as if they had never been committed, release from bondage or imprisonment**

2. What does the word "redemption" mean? (G629 – *apolytrosis*) **release because of payment of ransom; liberated, delivered**

3. The Greek for word for "forgiveness" is aphesis, which is the exact same word translated as **remission** in Matthew 26:28.

4. What does the word "authority" mean? (G1849 – *exousia*) **the power of influence and right privilege, the right to exercise power, must be obeyed or submitted to, ability or strength with which one is endued, which he either possesses or exercises**

5. What is the symbol of authority in law enforcement? **badge**

6. What does the word "power" mean? (G1411 – *dynamis*) **miracle working power, moral power, excellence of soul**

7. What is the symbol of power in law enforcement? **gun**

8. Say, "Father God, I hand you **(my pain, hurt, broken heart, guilt, condemnation, anger, bitterness, resentment, etc.)**

9. "What do you give me in exchange?" **Personal response from Father God directly to each person.**

Session 10
Fear Not, Only Believe

Foundation One

1. What were Jesus' words to Jairus right after hearing of his daughter's death? **"Do not be afraid; only believe, and she will be made well."**

2. What actions did Jesus take to lead Jairus out of fear and into faith? **He spoke in faith to Jairus to encourage Him. He permitted no one to go in except Peter, James, John, and the girl's parents. He spoke to the people, "Do not weep; she is not dead, but sleeping."**

3. What did Jesus leave to us as an inheritance? **Peace**

4. What does he command us in this scripture? **Do not let your heart be troubled or afraid!**

5. He gives us the **power** of the Holy Spirit.

6. He gives us the **love** of the Father.

7. He gives us **soundness of mind** from the Word of God, and Jesus is the Word made flesh. (John 1:14)

Foundation Three

#1 - Overcome fear by trusting God!

1. God's love is consummated within us through **union** and **communion** with Him.

2. The perfect love of God casts out **fear**.

3. When fear is cast out, faith is **given birth**.

4. Trust God. Don't try to figure out how to solve your concerns on your own. If fact, give up your right to **understand**!

5. It is **humbling** to give up self-control, and trust God to take care of your concerns.

6. What severe warning does this scripture give us? **Your adversary the devil walks about like a roaring lion, seeking whom he may devour.**

7. The enemy has been **defeated**, but not **destroyed**.

8. How do we resist the devil? **Remain steadfast in faith -- rooted, established, strong, immovable and determined.**

9. Fear is **deceiving**. Faith is **receiving**!

#2 - Overcome fear by taking fearful thoughts captive. Don't give them life through worry.

1. We are fully qualified to carry out **spiritual warfare** that overthrows and destroys the stronghold of fear.

2. What does the word "refute" mean? (G1869 – *epairo*) **Prove to be false by providing evidence.**

3. What are we to refute? **Anything that does NOT agree with God's Word.**

4. What does the word "captive" mean? (G163 – *aichmalotizo*) **Kept in confinement**

5. What does the word "obedience" mean? (G5218 – *hypakoe*) **Submission, compliance**

6. What are we to do INSTEAD of worrying? **Pray and give thanksgiving!**

7. What does God tell us to meditate on? **Things that are true, things that are of a good report, things that are praiseworthy!**

#3 - Overcome fear by guarding your speech.

1. How does the fruit in your life relate to your words? **Words of "death" produce the fruit of "death". Words of "life" produce the fruit of "life".**

2. Ask yourself, am I magnifying **God** and His Word, or am I magnifying the **problem**?

3. What is God's grave warning for us regarding double-mindedness? **For let not that man suppose that he will receive anything from the Lord.**

#4 - Overcome fear by using the "waiting room time" in a positive way.

1. Who is the author of your faith, and who brings it to completion? **Jesus!**

2. If you are questioning your level of faith, or questioning if you are doing enough praying or enough reading of the bible, or enough going to church – your focus is on the wrong person – yourself. This mindset is actually a hindrance to your faith, causing it to **slip away**.

3. BUT, if your focus is on Jesus and all that He has completed, once and for all for you, your faith **rises up**!

4. Does God give us trials or temptations? **NO!**

5. What happens within us as a result of going through trials? **Grow in spiritual maturity**

6. The "waiting room time" can be a time of immense spiritual **growth** and **inner** healing!

7. Often the **inner** person is transformed by the Holy Spirit before the manifestation of healing is seen on the **outer** person.

8. What does that look like? **Spend your time reading the Word, meditating on His promises for you, praising Him, listening to good teachers of the Word, etc.**

9. Whatever you feed on the most will **predominate** in your life.

#5 - Overcome fear by surrounding yourself with like-minded believers who will stand in faith with you.

1. What does it mean to agree? **To harmonize together, to believe the same truth!**

2. Establish a spiritual **mentor**, whom you can call any time that fear is attacking your faith. Don't hesitate to call your mentor to stand with you against the attack of the enemy.

3. Join a **small group** with whom you can study and discuss God's Word, pray in agreement, and stand united in faith.

4. Join a **church** whose doctrinal beliefs and actions agree with God's Word.

5. Sympathy agrees with the problem, and **nourishes** it.

6. Compassion agrees with God, and **strengthens** the receiver.

#6 - Overcome fear by praising and worshipping God!

1. He was **strengthened** in faith.

2. He did not waver in **unbelief**.

3. He was fully convinced that what God had **promised** He was also able to perform!

4. As we continually offer God our praise; as we magnify and exalt His holy name, He hears us, and delivers us from all of our **fears**.

INDEX

Abba 118-119
abide 58, 81, 102
Abraham and Sarah 44-45, 49, 52, 84-85, 146
agree 72, 73, 132-135, 145-146
angry 98, 111
author of confusion 73
author of faith 76, 141, 144, 148
authority 10, 12, 41, 46, 114, 122, 124, 127-129, 140-141, 149, 181, 182, 187
baptism of the Holy Spirit 90-92, 180
bitterness 103, 108, 110-111, 115, 126
body 20, 77, 123, 125, 132
boundaries 113
broken-hearted 17, 125, 131, 132
cancel 19, 108, 116, 120, 143
cast off 127, 128-129
causes for sickness and disease 32-35, 37
celebrate God's goodness 66, 78, 88, 135
centurion 19, 28, 40-41
child-like faith 44, 46-54
choose life 35, 69, 134
compassion 71, 72, 74, 134, 145, 147
concordance 16, 61, 63, 83
condemnation ... 116-118, 120, 124, 126, 129
confess 64-65, 113-114, 134, 179
confusion 73-74, 133
consequences of sin 97, 103-104, 123
consistency 73-74
debt 19, 99, 108-109, 110, 112, 115, 116, 126, 131

default operating system 68-73
disappointment 78
discouragement 78, 134-136
disobedience 34
divine healing 32, 52, 60, 185
double-mindedness 143-144
dynamis 91, 127
emotional dysfunction 124
emotional freedom 112-115, 126-127
emotional healing 75
emotions 122, 132, 134-138
enemy 33, 68-74, 98-100, 110-111, 122-128, 141-146
expectation 44, 88-89
faith 55-60
fall of man 33
fear 139-152
feed your heart 66, 77-78
focus on Jesus 71, 74, 76-77, 135, 144
forgive others 104-105, 108-111, 129
forgive yourself 116-120, 129
forgiveness of sin 19, 23-26, 99
free will 32, 81, 96, 113, 134
Gentile 39-40
godly living 93-105
God's perfect will 32, 58, 64
God's permissive will 32
grace 24-25, 40, 64-66, 118, 120
guard your speech 143
guard your heart 69, 72
healing of individuals 28-29

healing of multitudes 29-31
health 60, 61, 123, 132
holiness 95-96
hope 44
hope deferred................................. 134-135
humility 46-47
idolatry 37
infirmity... 38-39
Jesus - reflection of the Father............31, 38
joy..50, 136-138
kingdom of God 124
knowledge..............................33, 80, 87-88
law 35, 95, 104, 116-120
logos.. 57
love 80-81, 87-90, 104-105, 118-119, 141
manifestation............................. 75, 89-90
medicine 60-62
meditate.. 62-63, 68
mental dysfunction 124
mercy.. 39-40, 117
New Covenant................................99, 118
obedience 49-50, 122
offense 110-111
Old Covenant................................... 98, 118
oppressed 33, 126
peace 16-17, 59, 78, 135
power................59, 69, 91, 117, 124, 127, 141
praise and worship 77, 84-86, 146
prayer 56, 83-84
prayer of agreement 72, 145
pride 46-47, 120
prophecy... 18
prosperity.. 123
psychosomatic............................... 103, 125
rapha 17
reading the bible 83
reconciliation 108, 113, 118

redemption 33, 99, 108-109
relational healing 76
relationship with God........................ 80-90
remission 99, 108, 127
renewing of mind 65, 133
repentance 99-100
research.. 70-71
rhema 57-58
righteousness 23, 95, 97, 99
salvation................... 20-21, 23-26, 123
sanctification................................. 97, 98
sanctify 96
satan 33-34, 111, 116, 140-141, 148
sin 33-34, 94-95, 98-100, 103-104 118, 120, 123-124
soul 97-98, 122
soul wound 121-138
sowing and reaping................................ 35
sozo 20-21, 64, 125
speak words of life 69
spirit 122, 132
spiritual healing 75
staying balanced............................. 64-66
surrender.. 47
sympathy 71-72, 145
theology............................... 35, 41, 49
tongues 92, 180
transformed 65, 82, 133
traumatic event 124
trust 48-49, 80, 141-142
unforgiveness................... 103, 108-114
unworthy 116-120
waiting room 75-78, 144-145
worry 62, 68, 103, 133, 141-143

RECEIVING SALVATION

Have you surrendered your heart and your life completely to God? Have you received the salvation purchased for you through the shed blood of Jesus? Going to church does NOT ensure your salvation! Salvation is NOT inherited as part of your family background or culture! Living a "good life" does NOT guarantee your salvation either! It is with our heart that we believe and surrender all to Him. But the Word also says that we must use our mouth to invite Jesus into our life and to confess "Jesus is my Lord"!

If you have never taken this awesome step of faith, please stop right now and invite Jesus into your life. I'm including a simple prayer of salvation if you want to use it. Read it out loud with utter sincerity. Or just talk to God directly from your heart. The exact words aren't important. But your salvation IS more important than words can possibly say. It is your redemption from sin, sickness, and poverty. It is your eternal life!

Heavenly Father, I believe Your Word that says, "Whosoever shall call on the name of the Lord shall be saved" and "If you confess with your mouth the Lord Jesus, and believe in your heart that God has raised Him from the dead, you shall be saved" (Acts 2:21; Romans 10:9). You said my salvation would be the result of Your Holy Spirit giving me new birth by coming to live in me (John 3:5-6,14-16; Romans 8:9-11).

Father, I'm asking You now for salvation; for new birth. I desperately want You and need You in my life. I believe with all my heart that Jesus is Your Son and that He died on the cross for me. I am sorry for my sins, Lord God. Please forgive me for them and create a clean heart in me. I open the door of my heart and say, YES, I receive Jesus as my Savior, and I choose to follow Him as the Lord of my life!

Father, I surrender to You completely, with all of my heart and soul. I surrender my health to You. I surrender my mind, my will, and my emotions to You. Grow me up strong, Father, from the inside out. I hunger for completeness through You. I trust You, Lord, with all of my heart, and I relinquish control of my life to You. I declare that I am Your child, and that I will obey You as my heavenly Father.

I thank You, my Father, for Your love so great, so precious, that You have provided for me a life of abundance. I reach out to You, Lord, and receive all that You have planned for me! And I praise You, Who are so worthy to be praised! I love You more than words can possibly express. And You love me!

I declare that right now I am a child of God. I am free from sin and full of the righteousness of God. I am saved in Jesus' name! Amen! Glory be to God!

RECEIVING THE BAPTISM OF THE HOLY SPIRIT

Are you hungry to progressively become more deeply and intimately acquainted with Jesus, the Lord of your life? (Philippians 3:8) Are you longing to have deeper revelation of the Word of God? (John 14:26) Do you desire the anointing of the Holy Spirit to speak through you to others? You need the baptism in the Holy Spirit! Revelation knowledge is just one of the awesome benefits of receiving the baptism in the Holy Spirit. And your heavenly Father wants to give you the supernatural power you need to live this new life, and to take His Word into the world! (Acts 1:8) If you haven't already done so, I encourage you to receive this Promise – the baptism in the Holy Spirit – right now! (Luke 24:49)

All you have to do to receive the baptism in the Holy Spirit is to ask, believe, and receive. *For everyone who asks receives, and he who seeks finds, and to him who knocks it will be opened … how much more will your heavenly Father give the Holy Spirit to those who ask Him!* (Luke 11:10, 13b)

Go ahead and pray from your heart something like this:

> Father, Your Word says that the Holy Spirit is a gift. I do not have to work for it. All I need to do is ask and receive it. So I ask You, Jesus, come and baptize me with the Holy Spirit. I desire Your impartation in every part of my life. Lord, I want to receive all that You have for me!
>
> My heart cry is for a radical transformation in my walk with You. Consume me, O God, with Your holy fire! I receive, right now, as an act of my will and my faith, the baptism of the Holy Spirit.

In the book of Acts, everyone who was baptized in the Holy Spirit spoke in tongues. Speaking in tongues is totally biblical, and is your outward evidence of your inward filling! (Acts 2:1-4; 10:44-46; 19:6) Syllables from a language you don't recognize will rise up from your heart to your mouth. You must supply your voice and speak out your heavenly language. As you speak the spiritual words out loud by faith, you're releasing God's power from within and building yourself up in the spirit! (Jude 1:20) You can do this whenever you like!

Continue to speak forth in your heavenly language. Do not allow the enemy to tell you that you can't pray in tongues, because you can! Hallelujah! Continue to thank the Lord, to pour out your love for Him, to worship Him. Magnify Him with your heavenly language!

GOD'S MEDICINE
DECLARATIONS FOR HEALING AND DIVINE HEALTH

The following declarations are not direct quotations from the Bible. They are paraphrases of the referenced Scriptures, and faith statements based upon God's promises!

Healing

Sickness, you are cursed! You must flee! You can't exist in me. The Spirit of God is upon me and the Word of God is within me. Sickness, pain, fear, and oppression have no power over me for Gods' Word is my confession. (Mark 11:23)

Jesus said, "Every plant not planted by my heavenly Father will be rooted up." Disease, God has not planted you in me. Therefore, you must be rooted out of my body now, in Jesus' name. (Matthew 15:13)

Any cell or tissue that does not support life in my body is cut off from its life source. I command disease to dry up at the roots, in the name of Jesus. I command the seed of the root of disease to die, in the name of Jesus. My immune system will not allow disease to live in my body. It will wither and die at the roots, just like the fig tree that Jesus cursed! (Mark 11:20-24)

Jesus gave me the authority to use His name. That which I bind on earth is bound in heaven and that which I loose on earth is loosed in heaven. Therefore, I bind sickness and disease; you are evicted from my body and cast out into the sea. I loose the healing power of God in my body now, in Jesus' name. (Matt. 18:18)

Heavenly Father, as I give voice to Your Word, the law of the Spirit of life in Christ Jesus makes me free from the law of sin and death. And your Life is energizing every cell of my body. (Romans 8:2)

The same Spirit that raised Jesus from the dead dwells in me, permeating His life through my veins, sending healing throughout my body. (Romans 8:11)

In Jesus' Name, I forbid my body to be deceived in any manner. Body, you will not be deceived by any virus or disease germ. Neither will you work against life or health in any way. Every cell of my body supports life and health. (Matthew 12:25)

My immune system grows stronger day by day. I speak life to my immune system. I forbid confusion in my immune system. The same Spirit that raised Christ from the dead dwells in me and quickens my immune system with the life and wisdom of God, which guards the life and health of my body. (Romans 8:11)

Body, I speak the Word of Faith over you. I demand that every internal organ perform a perfect work, for you are the temple of the Holy Ghost. Therefore, I charge you in the name of the Lord Jesus Christ, and by the authority of His holy Word to be healed and made whole in Jesus' Name. (Proverbs 12:18)

I am not moved by what I see. I am not moved by what I feel. I am not moved by doctor's reports. I am moved only by what the Word says. By the stripes of Jesus, I am healed and made whole! God says it. I believe it. That settles it! (Acts 17:28, 1 Peter 2:24)

Divine Health

No unbelief or distrust will cause me to waver or question God's promise of healing. I am fully satisfied and assured that God is able and mighty to keep His Word and to do what He has promised! (Romans 4:20-21)

O Lord, my God, I cried unto You, and you healed me! Many are the afflictions of the righteous: but the Lord delivers me out of them all. There is no sickness or disease that can live in my body. By Jesus' stripes I am healed and walk in divine health every day of my life! (Psalm 30:2; Psalm 34:19)

My son (or my daughter), attend to My words, incline your ear unto my sayings. Let them not depart from your eyes; keep them in the midst of your heart. For they are life to those who find them, and health to all their flesh. I keep God's Word in my heart, and it is healing me all the time. It gives me long life and health. I'm so glad I'm healed. Thank you, Jesus, for setting me free and healing me! (Proverbs 4:20-22)

Jesus is the same yesterday, today, and forever. Jesus healed my body once and for all! I am forever healed and completely restored to normal! (Hebrews 13:8)

So then, Beloved, consecrated and set apart for God, you who share in the heavenly calling, thoughtfully and attentively consider Jesus, the Apostle and High Priest Whom you confessed as yours when you embraced the Christian faith! For in Him you live and move and have your being! (Hebrews 3:1; Acts 17:28)

Sickness and disease have no right to my body. They are a thing of the past for I have been delivered from the authority of darkness. (Colossians 1:13-14)

Father, I put you in remembrance of your Word, stating my case before you, holding fast to my confession of faith, without wavering, for you are faithful. I release my faith now and declare that I am the healed of the Lord. By the stripes of Jesus, I have been healed. (Isaiah 43:25-26; Hebrews 10:23; 1 Peter 2:24; Exodus 15:26)

My child, don't be afraid of recurring sickness or disease. I will continue to fight for you, just as I did when I first healed your body of sickness before your very eyes. You saw how I carried you, the way a Father carries His child. I will continue to go ahead of you on your journey. (Deuteronomy 1:29-31)

If you diligently obey the voice of the Lord your God, He will cause your enemies who rise against you to be defeated before your face; they shall come out against you one way and flee before you seven ways! (Deuteronomy 28:1a; 7)

Bless the Lord, O my soul; And all that is within me, bless His holy name! Bless the Lord, O my soul, and forget not all His benefits. You have forgiven all my iniquities; You have healed all my diseases; You have redeemed my life from destruction; You have crowned me with loving kindness and tender mercies; You have satisfied my mouth with good things so that my youth is renewed as the eagle. (Psalm 103:1-5)

Those who hope in the Lord will soar on eagle's wings. They will run and not grow weary. They will walk and not grow faint. (Isaiah 40:31)

Lord, You have blessed my food and my water, and you've taken sickness away from me. Therefore I will fulfill the number of my days in divine health. (Exodus 23:25-26)

Fighting Fear

I declare that I am strong, and the word of God (who is Love) lives in me. I overcome the evil one. I am an overcomer. (1 John 2:14; 1 John 4:4)

Peace I leave with you; My peace I now give to you. Not as the world gives do I give to you. Do not let your heart be troubled, neither let it be afraid. Stop allowing yourself to be agitated and disturbed; and do not permit yourself to be fearful and intimidated and cowardly and unsettled. Fear, you leave me now in the name of Jesus Christ of Nazareth. I have the peace of God in my mind and body. I refuse to worry or to be uptight about anything. Thank You, Jesus, for Your peace and love that I have on the inside of me. I am carefree, worry-free, burden-free, and anxiety-free in Jesus' name. (John 14:27)

I will rejoice in the Lord; I will exult in the victorious God of my salvation! The Lord God is my strength, my personal bravery, and my invincible army; He makes my feet like hinds' feet and will make me to walk (not stand still in terror, but to walk) and make spiritual progress upon my high places of trouble, suffering, or responsibility! (Habakkuk 3:18-19)

For God has not given me a spirit of fear; but of power, and of love, and of a sound mind. I present myself; spirit, soul, and body to my Heavenly Father in the name of Jesus. I command the spirit of fear, in the name of Jesus, by the POWER of the Holy Spirit, LEAVE ME NOW! Get away from me! Get out of my room! Get away from my family! Fear does not come from

God. So I rebuke fear from my mind and body in Jesus' name. I have the spirit of power, love, and a sound, disciplined mind. I have the mind of Christ. Thank you, Jesus, for setting me free. (2 Timothy 1:7)

Be anxious for nothing, but in everything by prayer and supplication, with thanksgiving, let your requests be made known to God; and the peace of God, which surpasses all understanding, will guard your hearts and minds through Christ Jesus. Finally, brethren, whatever things are true, honest, just, pure, lovely, and a good report; if there is any virtue (anything good), and if there is anything praiseworthy, think on these things. I refuse to be upset, worried, anxious, fearful, or uptight about anything. I will only think on those things that are true, honest, just, pure, lovely, and a good report. I will only think on positive things, in the name of Jesus. My mind is peaceful, quiet, healed and strong, because I have the mind of Christ. Thank You, Jesus, for healing my mind. (Philippians 4:6-8)

Declaring the Wonderful Works of the Lord

Nothing, nothing is as important to me as the priceless privilege of knowing Christ Jesus my Lord and of progressively becoming more deeply and intimately acquainted with Him. (Philippians 3:8)

I trust in the Lord with all my heart, and lean not on my own understanding. In all my ways I acknowledge Him, and He directs my paths. (Proverbs 3:5-6)

My eager desire and persistent expectation and hope, is that with my utmost freedom of speech and unfailing courage, Christ will be magnified and get glory and praise and be boldly exalted through me! (Philippians 1:20)

I pray that freedom of utterance may be given me, that I may open my mouth to proclaim boldly the mystery of the good news (the Gospel), for which I am an ambassador. I pray that I may declare it boldly and courageously, as I ought to do. (Ephesians 6:19-20)

I shall live and not die and I will declare the works of the Lord! (Psalm 118:17)

ALSO BY CINDY COX

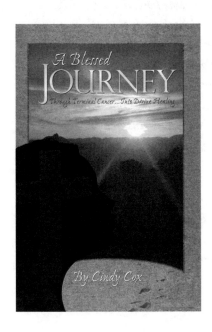

A Blessed Journey: Through Terminal Illness … Into Divine Healing is Cindy's true story. In the prime of her life, she was diagnosed with Stage 4 melanoma cancer, given six to nine months to live by the established medical community – and was then miraculously healed. In her testimonial book, Cindy tells of the journey she took as she was diagnosed with cancer, turned her life over to Christ and received her divine healing through faith. Cindy also addresses many difficult questions associated with divine healing:

- Is God's healing available for you too?
- How can you develop your faith to believe and receive your healing?
- What may stand in the way of receiving divine healing?
- Why do bad things happen to good people?
- Why are some people healed, but not others?

I have felt like I am living under the cloud of "cancer will come back, it's only a matter of time", since I had it in 2003. With the help of your book, I am claiming Jesus' healing power and am accepting His complete healing; believing now that cancer truly is over in my life! Thank you for being His messenger!
– Sue Kwant

This book changed my life! I suffered from migraines that numbered anywhere from 3-15 a month. Through learning what the Bible says about healing, changing the words that came out of my mouth and growing my faith, I am living free of headaches. The author presents the how-to's of healing and backs it all up scripturally, so even if you're like me, who in the beginning was skeptical, after you see it in the Word, you can only believe it. It couldn't be any more clear. – Amazon Review

I first read this book for myself a couple of years ago. My eyes were opened to the truths that were available for me regarding my own healing. The author's writing style is conversational and she uses easy to follow steps. I wasn't struggling with any big illnesses, but I still enjoyed this book.

It wasn't until 1 1/2 years later that I came to fully witness the power that this book discusses. My husband was completely immobilized by a sudden manifestation of several back problems. We were at the end of our natural abilities, and medical doctors couldn't help him anymore because of other health issues that prohibited routine treatment. Long story short, I read this book to him chapter by chapter at his bedside and our hopelessness changed to belief that healing would manifest, and it did. Miraculously, my husband's pain left in one moment and he was back to work in a matter of days, after being on his back in bed in immense pain for weeks. His life and our family's lives have been transformed, not just physically, but spiritually. – Amazon Review

This is a too compelling a story not to be told. God has ordained this work, and given the inspiration to Cindy to write it. She has become a present day inspirational writer. I do not hesitate to put her in the company of Paul or Luke. This story has to be told or the rocks will cry out. Fast and pray and seek God's divine direction, but above all tell the story! – Darryl Foster

ALSO BY CINDY COX

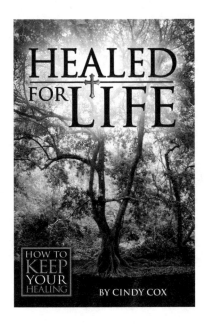

Healed For Life: How to Keep Your Healing

How do you keep your healing? How do you keep from living in fear of recurring disease? How do you go about walking in divine health all the days of your life? Living out a life of health in body, soul, and spirit requires a consistent and intimate relationship with the Healer. It requires a healthy spiritual "diet". It requires continual spiritual cleansing. If the disease attempts to resurface, it includes ridding yourself of fear, which is the opponent of faith. And it requires healthy living … good health habits, maintaining a stress and worry-free lifestyle, and keeping balance within your life. **Healed For Life** will provide you with clear and loving guidelines in how to consistently seek God first in every area of your life, and receive His ongoing benefits!

⁂

I can't say enough about this writer. Love her books. I bought two by this author. Really makes you think about LIFE! Very good read! Definitely would buy more books from her! LOVE IT! – Amazon Review

Healed for Life helped me understand clearly how to keep my healing and to help me recognize things that might come to steal it away from me. If you want all the benefits that God has for you for your life, this book will help you! I'm so grateful for the information and the dedication of the author to educate about God's will to heal! – Denise Baum

Healed For Life is clear and concise with everything in it being supported by Scripture. Cindy points out the significance that faith plays in receiving and keeping our healing. She also reminds us to seek the Healer, not the healing and the importance of keeping God at the center of our life in order to maintain our healing. In the second part of her book, Cindy discusses the subtle ways the enemy tries to steal our healing. She equips us with the necessary tools to defeat Satan and explains the power and authority we have over him in order to keep our healing. This book was extremely helpful for me, and I consider it a must read. – Kathy Bandol

CONTACT AND ORDERING INFORMATION

*Order books, read testimonies, download podcasts,
invite Cindy, and view her event schedule at:*

JesusChristHealsToday.com

*We would like to hear from you!
For prayer requests,
to share your own healing testimony,
or for further information about this ministry,
please contact Cindy via e-mail at:*

info@JesusChristHealsToday.com